AIP Diet

The Ultimate Guide for Intense Healing, Sparkling Health That Manages Autoimmune and Inflammation Disorders

Terrell Blaylock

Table of Contents

Introduction

Stop! Wait! Before you run for the hills, I urge you to take a deep breath and take a look at what I have to say. If you still feel the way you do then I will release you.

When you see or hear the word 'diet' in a title or an advertisement campaign, you are hesitant to go any further. I understand where you are coming from. The health and fitness markets are saturated with hundreds of different types of diets. While I am hesitant to use the little four-letter word that conjures up visions of authoritative figures wagging their fingers at your choice of food, we need to establish that diet or not, this is about a lifestyle – your lifestyle.

This book is going to help with an understanding of what goes on inside your body, and why your body has staged a coup d'état against you. Are you looking for alternative ways to manage the autoimmune disorders that have you doubled over in pain? Are you done with the food sensitivities that cause your condition to flare up and become unmanageable? Of course, you are.

No one is going to tell you to stop taking a medication that has been prescribed by a medical professional. You have been prescribed medication for a reason. While you think you can just sit back and let the medication do all the work, think about what you could be doing to help yourself. This is where I come in. I want to help you, by a process of elimination, pinpoint which foods you should be avoiding and/or eating more of to keep your condition at a comfortable level for you.

If you were thinking that this book was going to force you into a new age way of losing weight, are you not glad that you carried on reading? Not all diets are about losing weight. If you do end up losing a couple of pounds along the way, you may graciously accept the loss. This lifestyle is about reclaiming control over any and all debilitating side-effects that you might be experiencing by putting alternative measures in place. Autoimmune disorders are real. The pain and suffering is real.

Authoritative

Deciding to put pen to paper has taken many years of research to get to this point. Yes, I said years, as I have been researching nutrition and dieting, particularly concerning autoimmune disorders. I have been paying close attention to the effects certain foods have on people with various disorders, even seemingly healthy people. With everything that is going on in the world at present, I have decided that the time is right to share my knowledge. Every one of us needs to take care of the one body we have. We all have a choice. No one can tell you what to do. I strongly believe that if you are equipped with the right knowledge, you too will be able to make informed decisions based on what is best for your health.

Let us just get the elephant out of the room. We are in the midst of a global pandemic that has taken the world by the horns. Everything and everyone is upside down. No one knows what is going to happen. All we are being told is to wear masks, wash our hands, sanitize, and quarantine. One thing that has been brought up a lot since the start is that, if you are medically compromised or suffer from any autoimmune disorders, you should be taking extra precautionary methods to remain safe.

I Know and Understand

During my research, someone reached out to me and told me their experience after being diagnosed with an autoimmune disorder. In the early 2000s, there was not a lot of information about autoimmunity. Even doctors and specialists were in the dark as to what was going on and put a name to a disorder. Oh yes, Doctor Google had a lot to say but not much concise information backed by medical research.

The young lady that reached out to me went on to tell me how her caregiver spent hours researching ways to help her from looking like a blimp. They cut sodium from her diet, no more crisps, buttery salty popcorn, and crackers. This went on for 12 years. This is the story of a little girl who grew up with an autoimmune disorder, and how she reclaimed her health and body by managing her diet.

Imagine a little girl, six years of age, being diagnosed with an autoimmune disorder that has her emotions running amok. She has been on a cortisone treatment over a period of eight years. During this time, she becomes swollen and ends up with a "moon face". The teasing and bullying that follows her around break down her self-confidence in more ways than is necessary. Lose weight. Eat less candy. Eat more fruit and vegetables. The more she explains that she eats a healthy diet, does not eat candy, does not drink sugary drinks, or stays far away from fast-food, the more she is tortured by friends and even family. Depression sets in. Self-harm. The list is endless until she takes control.

Over the course of eight years, this young lady has learned what she can eat without the fear of her body reacting negatively. Where she was once admitted to the hospital every six weeks for immunoglobulin infusions to keep her antibodies happy, she now has an infusion once every six to eight months. What did she do that helped her maintain her disorder? She eliminated foods, and adopted a new approach to what she eats and drinks. It is working for her, and if it can work for her, it can work for you. Today, this young lady is managing her condition, and she is thriving and doing activities she was previously prevented from doing. After years of pain and suffering, teasing, and being judged, she is now able to enjoy walking her dogs on the beach, participates in horse-riding events, and enjoys spending time with her friends.

I realize that not everyone is in the same position as this young lady, but I do know that everyone who is suffering from whatever condition or ailment, knows what it feels like to be teased, judged, discriminated against, and so many more hurtful actions.

Where to From Here?

This book is designed to mimic a roadmap of your autoimmune disorder journey. You will experience a bumpy ride with a few pit stops along the way. No matter where your journey takes you, we are in this together. You have me in the palm of your hand. I want to be able to help you come to terms with your diagnosis. I want to show you that a not so favorable diagnosis does not mean that you should be planning your funeral. You are not the first, and will not be the last to be diagnosed with an autoimmune disorder. While there are no cures, there are ways in which you can manage your condition and live a normal life. If life gives you lemons, go and make lemonade. You do the best you can with what you are given. Do not retreat into a corner and fade away. Do not ever give your disorder or any negative situation in your life the upper hand.

I am not going to tell you that the Autoimmune Protocol (AIP) diet is all sunshine and roses. As with every new lifestyle change, you will not notice a change overnight. It does not mean that it is not working, it just means you have to persevere. You might want to give up, throw in the towel, and go back to living in pain, but I am urging you to ride it out. You have nothing to lose. I have already mentioned that this will be a process of elimination and considering how many different food types we have at our disposal, this could take weeks, if not months.

I am all about being positive and finding the good in everything. I might be a little too optimistic, but after years of researching and looking into the various disorders, I am hopeful that the symptoms can be managed by tweaking our diets until scientists have found a cure. Anything is possible if you have a positive attitude. If you are concerned about anything relating to your health, contact your healthcare provider instead of consulting the internet. I want to equip you with the basic information that you will need to understand what is going on inside your body. This book is in no way meant to diagnose your condition. I will not be telling you to stop taking medication or start taking potions. This book is about a holistic approach to help you, and give you an insight into a possible management plan for your condition. Let us get going as we start this journey of discovery.

"As with many life-altering events, an autoimmune illness is almost guaranteed to cause you to re-evaluate your priorities." - Joan Friedlander

Chapter 1:

The Immune System

Our bodies are amazing structures. Regardless of what we look like physically, our bodies are structured in such a way that our vital organs each have a place in which they fit. No two people have the same body structure, which makes each person unique. Yes, there are ways in which we can strive to acquire the desired shape and form, but that is altering what you were born with. You were given your specific body when you were conceived. You had to grow into your body. Your body is tailored to fit you. I am not here to preach to you and tell you everything you already know about your body, but I am going to tell you that you are unique. There is just one of you. It is up to you to keep that legacy going.

The subject of immune systems, whether healthy or compromised has been the center of attention since the onset of the global pandemic that brought the world to a screeching halt. Suddenly everyone is talking about how people with weak and compromised immune systems should self-isolate, wear masks and sanitize. The importance of the immune system did not register with us until it became a hot topic for discussion in news reports, information from healthcare providers, scientists, researchers, and general conversations with friends, family, or strangers.

Our immune systems are unique to us. No two people have the same immune systems, nor do they have the same responses when their bodies are being attacked. We can look at our immune systems as being our personalized army that lives beneath the layers, in cavities, and deep in the trenches. They lay in wait until an intruder enters the space that they are protecting. Our army works overtime to fight the battles we cannot see. Let us pause and take a step back in time to when our immune systems were created.

Back to the Beginning

If you were thinking that you were born with an immune system, you would be half correct. During the third trimester of pregnancy, antibodies are transferred from mother to baby via the placenta. During childbirth, some of the mother's antibodies are transferred to the baby, giving it an immunity boost. A baby's immune system is not strong enough to withstand infections, thus they are susceptible to all illnesses.

During the first couple of weeks and months, the mother's immunity wears off as the baby produces its own antibodies. There are ways to protect the baby and give their immune systems a boost until they have been able to build up their own defensive army. It is important to remember that there is no discrimination or judgment of any kind from me. I have said it before and I will continue saying it, that every person is different. People's circumstances are different, as are their beliefs. I am sharing what I have found during my research, and I will remain neutral and respectful without favoring one over the other.

Breastfeeding

No matter where you go, or who you speak to, everyone has an opinion regarding breastfeeding. It is so easy to pass judgment over moms who do not or cannot breastfeed. Whatever their reasons or choices, we do not have the right to make them feel like they are less than perfect. We are living in an age where scientists and researchers have developed a formula to contain all the essential nutrients to mimic breast milk. No matter what the social media warriors or the opinionated neighbors down the street have to say, everyone has a right to make a decision that is best for them.

Immunizations

This is a section where one has to tread lightly, almost walking on hot embers. There is a lot of controversy surrounding immunizations or vaccinations. Again, every person is entitled to have their opinion. I am not here to reprimand you or judge you for your decisions. Most parents vaccinate their children up until their teen years, as well as playing catch-up if they were to miss any shots at their wellness checks. The standard immunizations protect against potentially life-threatening illnesses such as measles, polio, and certain types of meningitis.

Introducing Food

Diet plays an important role in building up and strengthening the immune system of the growing baby and child. Everyone seems to be on the fence about when to start feeding your baby solids, and what to start with. If you ask a pediatrician, they will give their recommendation based on the baby's growth chart. Most recommend introducing solids at around six months but it is a personal choice, especially when exclusively breastfeeding. When the baby starts eating solids, it is important to focus on a variety of nutrient-rich foods that will add vitamins and minerals to their diets so that they can start building up their army of defense against viral or bacterial infections.

Immune System Explained

As mentioned at the beginning of the chapter, the immune system is your own personalized army that has been designed to protect your body from the inside. The immune system consists of a network of cells and proteins that kill or ward off harmful intruders. These cells and proteins are known as antibodies and they protect our bodies from diseases, infections, and viruses.

You are exposed to millions of germs, viruses, fungi, parasites, and bacteria daily. Exposure happens in many ways such as touching, kissing, sneezing, coughing, talking, and so many more. We cannot be hiding in a bubble for the rest of our lives, which is why our immune systems work so hard to adapt to the ever-changing pathogens to which we are exposed. Countries throughout the world are adjusting to the new normal as their citizens wear masks when they go out in public. Do not view the wearing of a mask as a punishment, but rather as a lifesaver. Nothing is one hundred percent foolproof and yes, you can still be exposed to airborne pathogens while wearing masks, but at least there is a bit of protection.

The Function of the Immune System

You can think of your immune system as your personalized home security system. When an intruder enters your home, the alarm starts going off to alert the owners. This is what the immune system does, it defends our bodies against harmful infections and diseases. When our bodies come under attack, the immune system responds with guns blazing. Unfortunately, not all security systems are secure enough to block all intruders. Some sneak past the barricades and continue with their battle. As far as they go, the more resistance they will encounter. Battles tend to weaken the body, and the defenses are lowered which would require some additional assistance with the help of medication.

The immune system also faces attacks from the body when it accidentally alerts the antibodies of a harmless threat. The story about *The Boy Who Cried Wolf* in *Aesop's Fables* comes to mind. Each time the antibodies are dispersed for no reason, healthy antibodies come under attack which brings on a whole host of issues, such as allergic reactions and autoimmune disorders.

The Structure of the Immune System

Our immune systems consist of three layers of defense that protect and defend our bodies from various attacks. These attacks are presented in the form of germs, bacteria, or parasites, as well as metals and toxins. Each defensive layer serves a purpose in your body. As each layer is compromised, the foreign entities break through to the next layer until the threat is under control. No matter how well you take care of yourself, you will always be faced with challenges where your body and health are concerned.

We will be taking a closer look at the three layers that make up our immune systems. These layers are designed to keep our bodies safe from harmful entities. Each layer offers a specific, more complex line of defense that prevents our bodies from being overridden with illness, infection, and disease.

Barrier Immunity

The first layer of our immune system has been named, aptly, the barrier. Whatever harmful germs enter our bodies are met by the first responders.

Skin

Our bodies are covered by skin, which coincidentally, happens to be the body's largest and most important organ. The skin acts as a barrier that stops pathogens from entering our bodies. This is where we have to take a step back and show our skin appreciation, because of all it does and means to our health and well-being.

Our skin produces extra protection by way of chemical and biological barriers. The cells produce and secrete germicide which will repel and kill off potential invaders. Our skin also contains immune cells that offer protection against infection if harmful germs should enter through our skin by way of a cut, a pinprick, or a graze. Whichever way we look at it, our skin literally has us covered.

Respiratory System

The fine hairs found in the respiratory system, known as the respiratory cilia, moves in a way that flushes escort foreign entities out of your system. The respiratory cilia act as a physical barrier that protects your lungs from harmful bacteria. Smokers have a compromised barrier which increases your chances of suffering from chest infections. Germicides are present and active in the respiratory system in the form of mucus which aids the defense against infections.

Gastrointestinal System

The gastrointestinal system is protected by acids which consist of a low pH balance. These acids destroy potentially harmful microorganisms that you would consume. Our tears contain an antimicrobial protein called lysozyme that aids in killing off harmful pathogens. The more you cry, the better your chances are of flushing your body and protecting your immune system from harmful intruders.

Innate Immunity

If the barrier immunity is compromised and harmful bacteria slip through the cracks, they enter the innate immunity which is part of the immune system we are born with. The innate immunity is composed of cells which are white blood cells.

Neutrophils

Neutrophils make up a majority of the cells in the innate immune cells. They are the first responders who detect and destroy harmful pathogens. Neutrophils are also known as phagocytes. They recognize foreign entities and eat them before they can cause infections. The neutrophils also contain enzymes that put up a fight when harmful pathogens enter the bloodstream. They are able to absorb the pathogens when an infection breaks through the innate barrier.

Eosinophils

Eosinophils fight many cellular parasites and bacterial infections. These cells are vital in fighting certain infections. If there are too many eosinophils in the system, they do tend to create havoc with the immune system and cause tissue damage, which is responsible for allergies and certain inflammatory disorders, such as asthma.

Basophils

Although they consist of the least amount of white blood cells in the body, basophils are responsible for fighting parasite-type infections. Basophils aid the blood clotting process as they contain heparin. As with eosinophils, if there are too many basophils in the system, they too cause allergic reactions.

Additional Cells

There are many more cells within the innate immune system that serve to protect us. However, as we know, too much of a good thing is not always good and if good cells are abundant, they can cause various health issues such as allergies, inflammation, and various disorders.

- Mast cells

- Dendritic cells

- Monocytes

- Macrophages

- Natural killer cells

Adaptive Immunity

The third layer of the immune system is known as adaptive or acquired immunity. This part of the immune system is not present when we are born. The older we get, the stronger it becomes by being exposed to the various types of viruses, bacteria, or parasites.

Adaptive immunity comes into play when the barrier and innate immunities are compromised. It is made up of specialized cells known as lymphocytes. Each of these cells has a memory bank that remembers all foreign entities that it encounters. When an invader slips through the first two layers of the immune system, they are met by the lymphocytes or antibodies.

As they are new to the body, and not flagged as being potentially harmful, the cells will remember these pathogens. Repeat exposure of these entities will result in the cells remembering their initial introduction and the antibodies will contain and destroy them.

Role-Players of the Immune System

Every part of your immune structure has a specific function in your health and well-being. There are various 'checkpoints' in your body that prevent intruders from causing mayhem. You might have heard about these organs, tissues, or cells that call your body home, but never quite understood their function. Now is the time to give you a crash course on some of what forms part of the immune system.

Lymphatic System

The lymphatic system is a unique thoroughfare that is found throughout the body. The intricate system transports lymph throughout the body to cease and desist any foreign entities that have entered the bloodstream. Lymph is a milky fluid that contains white blood cells, our defense army, throughout the body to clear any debris, such as dead cells and lingering germs.

The lymph nodes, which form part of the lymphatic system, are little lumps that are found in the neck, armpits, and groin. Lymph nodes are early detectors and alert your body that there is a possible infection due to swelling and pain caused by colds or flu.

Bone Marrow

Bone marrow is a life-saving spongy substance inside your bones that is used to treat various diseases and cancers. The fatty bone marrow is important to the immune system as this is where your red and white blood cells are created.

Spleen

The spleen is very important to our bodies. It breaks down old red blood cells and preserves cells to be used for any future infections that could attack the body. It is possible to continue a normal, healthy life without a spleen, but it is important to take care of the organs you have.

In Summary

I will be reiterating that the human body is an amazing structure. Day in and day out, it is exposed to all kinds of germs, bacteria, parasites, and whatever pathogens are floating around. While we enjoy a carefree life, our immune systems are hard at work producing antibodies to ward off invaders, or mucous membranes to prevent illnesses or infections. Every compartment in our body holds a vital organ or protects a delicate muscle that is needed in the war raging deep within our bodies.

Sadly, not everyone has the luxury of having the freedom of sitting back while their army battles infections and diseases. Some have an immune system that does not work the way it should. Before you start pointing fingers and playing the blame game, we have to remember that no two people are the same. Some people are just wired differently. Some people do not have the defenses others do. For whatever reason, we show compassion and understanding.

In a world that is strife with hatred, anger, finger-pointing, and judgment, we need to stop and take stock of what is going on around us. No one knows what is going on in someone else. Outwardly they might look healthy, but under the layers is someone that is broken and struggling to keep everything together. Be careful of judging the book by its cover.

Chapter 2:

Autoimmunity

Growing up, we were entertained by stories told to us by our parents and grandchildren when they were growing up as carefree children. The stories would always begin with "When I was your age—". I recall tales of how they would walk for miles in rain, snow, wind, and rain to get to school. Sometimes they did not have the proper clothing or shoes to protect them from the harsh elements of nature. They ate food they grew on their property and drank freely from rivers and fountains. They survived to tell us their stories.

The world and the way we live in these modern times have changed dramatically. The more the population increases, and continues to increase, the more we rely on quick and easy. Technology joined the party and brought televisions, smartphones, gaming consoles, and many more conveniences. Fresh air and outdoor activities were replaced with interactive television games. The need to succeed took away the need for relaxation and self-care.

Wholesome cooking, canning, and baking was replaced with prepackaged meals, tin foods, and "quick and easy" out of the box baking. Life has become easy, erring on the side of caution by saying that it has made people lazy. Processed foods and drinks have a home in our pantries, food storage rooms, and refrigerators. It is less time-consuming stopping at a fast-food restaurant or popping a premade meal into the microwave than cooking a meal from scratch.

I will not knock our modern-day practices as they do have a purpose, but I do believe that a comparison between the 'olden' days and our current days will put our health concerns into perspective. Thanks to these modern-day practices, doctors, scientists, and researchers can identify conditions about our health and well-being more efficiently than 50 years ago. Thanks to all the research, some of our health concerns have names.

Autoimmunity Defined

In Chapter 1 we learned about the immune system and how it is structured. We know that there are three layers to our immunity; namely, the barrier, the innate, and the adaptive immunities. Each layer serves a purpose in keeping harmful entities under control. The adaptive or acquired immunity is made up of organs, proteins, and cells, and they are trained to recognize harmful entities. As previously mentioned, when pathogens break through the first and second barrier, they are flagged by the antibodies in the adaptive immunity.

As far as protection goes, we know that nothing is ever 100% secure. The same can be said for our immune systems. We might be taking multivitamins, exercising, and eating a healthy diet, but we still get sick. The antibodies in our system detect, contain, and destroy the intruders. Unfortunately, the immune system is not all that perfect and will be misled into thinking that the healthy cells are a threat. Autoimmunity is a battle of good versus good, and the antibodies start attacking healthy muscles, tissues, organs, and cells.

The Battle of Good Versus Good

You do not need a degree in medicine to understand autoimmunity. You want to understand what is going on in your body, and it is your right to ask as many questions as you want so that you can expand your knowledge. We already know that our adaptive immune system is something that is trained from the moment we are born. Training your immune system is something that cannot be planned or scheduled in advance. The training begins when you are exposed to germs, bacteria, or parasites. A line of defense is built up during our formative years when we receive the necessary nutrients from our feedings, vaccinations that were administered, and eventually the food to which we were introduced. The building up of the immune system does not happen overnight.

We build up our antibodies as we are introduced to everyday life, people we encounter, playing at the park, or eating at restaurants. No matter where you go, you will be exposed to germs and bacteria. This is all part of life. We know that we have to wash our hands regularly but all it takes is a little droplet of saliva, contaminated food or even kissing your partner for germs to sneak their way into your bloodstream. The antibodies stand guard for such instances and they are ready to identify, contain, and destroy the intruders.

It seems insane that our seemingly healthy internal organs, muscles, tissues, or joints are being attacked and destroyed by the very thing that is meant to keep us healthy. There are no simple explanations as to why this happens. Some people have an overactive immune system that is easily triggered if it suspects danger. The danger, in this instance, is an overabundance of antibodies that could be viewed as threats due to their rapid growth and insurgence within our bodies. We could almost say that the antibodies are trigger happy and go around with guns blazing so that they can be praised for doing a good job. Unfortunately, the eager beavers are identifying healthy organs, muscles, and tissues as threats and they are causing more harm than good.

Key Contributors to Autoimmunity

Autoimmunity has been part of you since the day you were born. Yes, it had to be trained over the years. The training never ends, especially with all the different types of pathogens we are exposed to daily. Every moment of every day, your autoimmunity is fighting to ensure you do not succumb to infections, whether viral or bacterial. We know what happens when good battles good, and thus it seems only fitting to introduce you to your army. This army is responsible for the makeup, breakup, and destruction of your immune system.

Lymphocytes

Lymphocytes are white blood cells that have a role in fighting infections in our bodies. The white blood cells originate from the bone marrow where they are produced and sent out to search for harmful pathogens. The lymphocytes are broken up into two different cells namely the B lymphocytes and T lymphocytes.

B Lymphocytes

The function of the B lymphocytes is to recognize antigens. The B lymphocytes are released into the bloodstream from the bone marrow and make their way to various organs and tissues such as the spleen, lymph nodes, and tonsils. Each of these B cells is equipped with receptor cells or effector cells that will connect with antigens. When the antigen connects with the receptor cells, they become part of the B lymphocyte.

The B lymphocytes will break down the antigen. The spoils of the breakdown settle on the surface of the B lymphocyte. Each antigen that enters our bodies goes through the same process in order to recognize them and build up a defense for future attacks. These are broken down antigens are transformed into plasma cells that produce antibodies. Each plasma cell is specific to the antigen that was initially identified by the receptors.

T Lymphocytes

T lymphocytes or T cells are broken into three different sections which each has a functional role in what it does in your body.

- Cytotoxic T Cells

Much like the B lymphocytes, cytotoxic T cells have receptors on their surfaces that recognize invaders on the surface of the infected or compromised cells. It will envelop the cell and discharge cytotoxins that will kill cells that have previously been flagged as antigens.

- Helper T Cells

As the name suggests, these cells help the white blood cells by recognizing antigens and alerting the B lymphocytes and T Lymphocytes of a potential threat.

- Regulatory T Cells

Regulatory T cells are responsible for suppressing the immune system from being overenthusiastic in the way it responds to the threat of danger. These cells are important to our immune systems as they prevent the white blood cells from attacking antigens that are already identified and essential to our immune responses.

Autoantigens/Self-Antigens

Autoantigens/self-antigens are a normal occurrence in our bodies. They are a part of our makeup which helps the immune system by producing antibodies to combat harmful pathogens. Antigens are round up by B cell receptors and are broken down to determine whether they are friend or foe. The cells will remember the action taken and will react accordingly. Autoantigens/self-antigens help the immune system by keeping up with what is going on deep within our bodies.

Autoantibodies

We know how antibodies are created with the help of the B lymphocytes, and we know that they are there to fight off harmful pathogens that creep in through the adaptive immunity or the third layer of our immune systems. As previously mentioned, sometimes the antibodies are a little too eager to protect our bodies and they will identify threats that are not threats. When these eager antibodies get riled up, they start viewing threats that are healthy and attack the tissues, muscles, organs, the blood, and organs. These types of antibodies are known as autoantibodies.

Contributing Factors Leading to Autoimmunity

You have been presented with so much information about your immune system and its ability to keep you healthy. You know about the antibodies that are fighting a battle against foreign entities deep within your body. Why are your antibodies, those plasma cells that are custom-made for your body, attacking your healthy organs, tissues, or muscles? You have spent hours, if not weeks and months, doing independent research to gain some clarity about autoimmune disorders. No one can give you a satisfactory answer without repeating everything we have already mentioned here. All you want to know is what causes autoimmune disorders. Did you do something wrong to have been diagnosed with one of the many disorders? Why is it so difficult to get a straight answer out of someone without the whole repetitive spiel?

While many believe that the reason for illnesses or disorders is poor self-care, hygiene, or diet, this is and stays their opinion. The answer to your burning question about the causes of autoimmune disorders is that there are no definitive causes. Immunologists, epidemiologists, clinicians, and scientists do not have the answers. Research and testing is and has been a work in progress for decades, but due to the exposure of new viruses, bacteria, and parasites daily, it is difficult to come to a concrete conclusion. The possible causes could be speculated and hinted at, no one is certain why the antibodies take the action they do. We have to give the researchers and scientists credit for their perseverance and ongoing research, and we have to remain hopeful that they come up with the answers you and everybody else wants.

Having touched on the amount of research that has been performed, there are some unproven theories which we can look at. Please keep in mind that these theories regarding the possible causes have not been proven and are therefore not to be taken as gospel. Although no one knows what causes our antibodies to launch a full-scale war on our organs, researchers have documented some unproven theories collected by doing various studies on patients with different autoimmune disorders. It is worth mentioning that, to date, there are more than 90 autoimmune disorders that have been recorded, and they are on the increase, especially when a global pandemic is spreading like wildfire. According to various reports, the National Institutes of Health have given an estimation that 23.5 million Americans have been diagnosed as having an autoimmune disorder. We will be taking a look at a couple of the factors that could lead to developing an autoimmune disorder. In Chapter 4, we will be looking at various autoimmune disorders, as well as some of the risk factors that could potentially lead to a positive diagnosis.

Genetic Factors

Researchers have concluded that if someone in your family has an autoimmune disorder, you are at risk of inheriting that gene. This does not necessarily mean that your gene will be triggered, and it may remain dormant. It would be in your best interest to get yourself tested, as symptoms do not always present themselves. If detected early, you have the upper hand in that you can adopt a lifestyle change.

Environmental Factors

Due to the increase in population, the world has changed to accommodate its growing tribe. More factories are built, more motor vehicles are on the roads, and the dynamics have changed to adapt. As we are well aware, the year 2020 has brought about many challenges and changes. Some might believe that the world is punishing us. Others believe that it is just something that was meant to happen. Whatever you believe, it does not take away the fact that the world our parents and grandparents grew up in has evolved.

We are exposed to pollution daily, whether it be from the factories or our motor vehicles. These harmful emissions need to go somewhere. It is believed that the environment plays a role in our health and more people are being diagnosed with autoimmune diseases and cancer. A smoker might not think he is causing harm to anyone but himself, when in fact his secondhand smoke is more dangerous to those around him. Regulations have been put in place to stop smokers from smoking in public areas and confined spaces but there are those that do not care.

Water shortage is a real concern. Not only is the water drying up but pollution, such as an abundance of plastic, enters our reservoirs. This leads to our water dwellers being suffocated, rotting and the water becomes contaminated. We need water to survive. Water is essential to our health.

Lifestyle Factors

We have all heard that we need to eat healthy food, exercise daily, get sufficient sleep, not consume alcohol, and stop smoking. I am sure there are more examples but these are the most common. Autoimmune disorders do not have a time frame for when they develop. It does not matter if you are skinny or severely obese, if you have a pre-determined gene, it is your time to host.

This does not mean that one can go ahead and live a carefree life of partying, smoking, eating, and taking drugs. It cannot be stressed enough that if you look at what is going on around you and in the world, things are rapidly changing. There is a virus that has claimed the lives of millions and researchers are fighting against time to produce a vaccine. That is a work in progress and no one knows when that will happen. It is up to us, you and me, to protect our bodies.

Consider changing your habits. Change your lifestyle for the better. If you are obese, make some positive changes. Being obese could lead to inflammatory disorders, thyroid disease, or inflammatory bowel disease. Smokers should consider giving up the smelly habit. If you are a heavy smoker, wean yourself off until you have kicked the butt for good. Your lungs, microbiome, and family will thank you. Incorporate some exercise into your daily routine. You do not need a gym membership. Start by moving. Move away from the computer and do something physical like dancing or sweeping your house. Not only will it get the blood flowing, but it will also make you feel better. Anything is possible if you put your mind to it.

Gender

As you will see when you get to Chapter 4, more women than men are diagnosed with autoimmune disorders. This does not mean the men can breathe a sigh of relief, as genetics do still play a role.

In Summary

Our bodies and composition are amazing structures. They have the ability to do what no modern-day practice can do, and that is to build up and protect our organs, tissues, muscles, or joints. We have dug deep and explored our bodies from the inside out to understand how everything works without the information being overwhelming. As much as we hate to admit it, we have to appreciate the hard work our custom-made army does for us. No two people have the same defense structure or the same symptoms.

When our immune systems are compromised, whether it be from taking medication, eating food, or being in contact with someone who is ill, harmful pathogens will enter our bodies. Sometimes there are too many pathogens swimming around for the lymphocytes to identify quickly enough and a battle of wills starts. While the pathogens swim around and cause havoc, the autoantibodies kick in and start attacking their allies. When this happens, the good versus good battle, it paves the way for you to develop an autoimmune disorder.

Your immune system is hard at work trying to hold everything together and make sure everything works as it should. There is no proven evidence of why your antibodies turn on your internal organs, muscles, or joints. Maybe it is time for a total body revolution. Use the risk factors that are presented to us, whether mentioned here or not, and fight for what is good for us. Our world is governed by convenience, not really but in the context, you know what I am getting at. As humans, we want easy and straightforward. We have fast-food restaurants that make us a delicious, not so nutritious meal in minutes and we are oblivious to what is added. We have stores that sell us pre-packed meals that take minutes to heat and eat; we are oblivious to what is added.

Remember your parents and grandparents, and their carefree youth growing up without the modern technology and convenience. Their meals were prepared daily using fresh ingredients. They never needed a magnifying glass to read the fine print on the labels of cans, bottles, and boxes. Everything they put into their food was fresh and additive-free.

Take control of your life today. Let us fill our bodies with happy antibodies that do not fight anymore and where everyone gets along. By the end of this book, you are going to be excited that you decided to take control of your body and your health. We can all work together.

Chapter 3:

Myths and Misconceptions

Did you know that just about everybody on this earth is a doctor? Everybody with a computer, a tablet or a smartphone and an internet connection, that is. Yes, Doctor Google, Doctor Bing, and Doctor Yahoo have trained many couch doctors—without the practical training—to diagnose and treat just about every common and complex ailment, suggest some type of remedy, and concoct some potions to expel any disorder from your body. We cannot fault these well-meaning couch doctors. Their research probably came about while they were looking for information to help a loved one. No one wants to see someone they care about feeling despondent or in pain from whatever disorder they are plagued with.

The older generation stands ready with their old-wives tales to help get rid of the ailment. They have many "tried and tested" natural mixtures. They are quick to tell you that they cured someone of a terrible disease and how thankful that person is to have been given a new lease on life. Anyone with a molecule of respect in them will not want to argue with well-meaning people who just want to help. It is not easy to tell these people that you are skeptical to take anything without speaking to your immunologist or epidemiologist.

We know and understand that everybody wants to help, but it is important to know that what you read on blogs, websites, or watch on videos, should be taken with a grain of salt. I realize that you want to find a way to cure your disorder. I completely understand that you do not want to take medication that negatively impacts your life. You want and are willing to do and try just about anything to help you feel 'normal', even if it is not the smartest way to go about reclaiming your health.

Dangers of Myths

There are several well-meaning individuals out there, whether in real life or the cyber world. Everyone has a whole lot to say and consider themselves experts after reading journals or websites about certain health issues and challenges. I have previously mentioned that whatever you read or advice you are given needs to be taken with a grain of salt. What worked for Joe's skin condition might not work for Mary's. What helped Sarah's arthritis might help Eve's. No two people are the same and no two people will have the same reaction to medication or home remedies.

Several myths are circulating the internet, social media, and general media referencing the global pandemic we are experiencing. There are so many misconceptions and unfortunately, there are innocent victims that will fall prey to the misinformation. It is so easy to hide behind a keyboard, change your name, and add content to a blog or even as a comment to a post for myths to be noticed. Sometimes myths are taken out of context. Whatever the case, there are hundreds and thousands of myths relating to health and well-being. I am hoping to highlight the common misconceptions concerning some of the myths we have been told over the years. Some of these myths are as old as the hills and others have been 'thoughtfully' introduced as early as 2019.

Everyday Health Myths

I wanted to give you a broader view which highlights the various myths people are faced with daily. These are people that do not have major health concerns and present as healthy individuals. Unfortunately, they are targeted by people who are basing their knowledge (or lack thereof) on a person's appearance, skin tone, body definition, or type of food/drinks being consumed.

Food Deprivation

This is one that many have heard and have tried at some point during our lifetime. If you have a couple of stubborn pounds around the belly, you should not be eating anything that can contribute to weight gain. In other words, you are being told to eat non-nutritious low- to no-calorie foods. By doing this, you will lose those stubborn pounds in no time.

You should always eat a balanced meal. Do not starve yourself, as you will be causing your body distress. The way to lose weight is not by depriving yourself, but by eating what you want to in the correct portions. There are hundreds of diets that each offer their own perspective on what you should be doing to lose weight. If you want the right advice, visit your doctor who will refer you to a dietician for the correct portions.

Bottle Versus Tap Water

The bottle versus municipal water will be one of those where each person has an opinion. One person will say that the bottle is best and another will say that the water out of the tap is better. We have been brainwashed into believing everything we have been taught while growing up. Remember your parents and grandparents that grew up before there were different types of bottled water or flavors? They drank their water out of streams, brooks, and fountains, and they were fine.

Is a bottle better than tap? In my opinion, no. If you add up the process involved in making a single bottle of water, drinking straight from the tap is a better and healthier option. Ask yourself, where does that bottle come from? What process has it been through to mold it into a bottle? What happens when you are finished with that bottle? Do you recycle it or does it become part of the landfill?

I am in no way an environmentalist, I am just someone who cares about what I put into my body which can be in the form of fluid, food, or medication. Next time you visit Costco, Target, or Walmart, take your magnifying glass along so that you can read the fine print on the labels of the bottled water.

Energy Drinks

These drinks are more harmful than good. The millennials of our time live on energy drinks. They believe that there is some miracle additive that can keep you focused and going for 30 hours a day. No matter how many times you tell people that energy drinks are made up of caffeine and do not contain some superpower, the more you are met with arguments and 'facts' from the addicts.

If you want a healthier alternative than fueling your body with processed drinks, such as any one of the many energy drinks on the market, opt for the real deal. If you drink coffee, freshly ground by you, you know what you are getting. You also have control as to what you add to your drink.

Detox

Another one of those myths that have been fed through as being beneficial to your health. There are many different products on the market that aid in detoxing the body before embarking on a new diet or lifestyle. Detoxing involves anything from drinking supplements to drinking homemade brews.

The idea of detoxifying has many scratching their heads in confusion. We have kidneys and a liver that flush any toxins out of our body daily. We drink water, not only for hydration but to flush out harmful toxins. The whole idea around detoxing is a way for companies to make money off desperate people who want to lose weight.

Flu Shots

"If you do not want to get the flu, you need to get the yearly flu shot." This statement is one that is used every year. No matter where in the world you are, everyone has an opinion regarding flu shots. The common misconception is that when you get your yearly flu shot, you are being injected with the flu virus.

When you are administered the flu shot, you are not going to get sick because the flu shot does not contain an active virus. The reaction many people get after having the shot varies from having sore muscles, fevers, or headaches which mimic flu-like symptoms but it is not the flu. The best to do if you are feeling fluish, is to remain hydrated, eat nutritious meals, and get rest.

Sunblock

Sunblock should be part of everybody's morning ritual when getting ready for the day. Men and women should be starting the day with a healthy slather of sunblock, and continue reapplying it throughout the day. It does not matter whether the sun shines, it is pouring with rain or a blizzard, making use of sunblock should be like applying body lotion. It is never too late to start taking care of your body.

Essential Oils

Many people believe that essential oils are vitally important for health and wellbeing, some even being cures for certain diseases and ailments. Aromatherapy is not a new trend that has jumped onto the market and has been around for many years. There is no scientific evidence that proves that the use of essential oils will cure any diseases. However, there is proof that, if not used correctly or ingested, essential oils can be harmful.

Bleach

This is something that has thrown the medical world for a loop. There have been numerous reports from various sources claiming that drinking sodium chlorite solution, commonly known as bleach, will kill harmful pathogens. On any given day, bleach is an excellent disinfectant to be used in and around the home to sanitize and clean surfaces. This substance should not be ingested in any way, as it can cause your internal organs to shut down and could end your life.

If we look at the effect bleach has on our color clothing, you will notice that it almost instantly discolors your clothes. If your clothing is damaged within seconds of spilling some bleach, imagine what it would and could do to your organs. Love yourself enough to not listen to unfounded cures. Speak to your doctors, immunologists, or epidemiologists to guide you along the right path.

Internet

The information you might read on the internet might seem like the real deal, especially when accompanied by some 'facts'. It is easy to self-diagnose and administer some home- or holistic remedies that are given. It is best you err on the side of caution and get the real facts from someone who has studied and trained in the medical field. Doctor Google, Doctor Bing, or Doctor Yahoo have the knowledge base that millions of users have submitted. What worked for others might not work for you and, as in the case of the bleach scenario, you could end up doing more harm than good.

Autoimmune Health Myths

We have a general understanding of how society perceives what we should be doing to ensure we live a long and healthy life by offering their views. These views are not necessarily the views of trained medical professionals and should not be taken seriously. If you have specific questions that have not been mentioned in this chapter, make up your list and contact your doctor instead of turning to uninformed sources.

We have covered some of the everyday myths we are faced with. We will be moving along to take a look at some of the common myths around having an autoimmune disorder. When you tell people that you have an autoimmune disorder, they put you under a microscope to scrutinize your health or actions. You can share your knowledge of your condition with people, but you will still be under the spotlight.

No Immune System

This is one of the first things people think of when you mention that you have an autoimmune disorder. We have to keep reminding people that everyone is born with an immune system. Some people, however, have problems with their adaptive immune systems in that they do not work the same way a healthy person does. Having an autoimmune disorder means that you are wired a little differently and your immune system shorts itself which leads to your antibodies fighting against themselves.

Looks Can Be Deceiving

You might look perfectly healthy but that does not mean that you are physically healthy. Not all sick people look and act the same. No one will ever know what is going on within your body or that of someone with an autoimmune disorder. The same can be said for someone that suffers from depression. Someone might look happy, is smiling and making jokes, but deep within their souls, they are fighting a soul-destroying disease. Many examples can be used but until you know a person and what they are faced with, be compassionate instead of judging them based on their outward appearance.

Weight

It is easy for the judgmental Judy to assume that because someone is built or structured differently, that all it will take is a miracle cure, such as dropping some pounds, to be cured. If this was the case, there would be stick figures inhabiting this earth. As it stands, there are autoimmune disorders that contribute to weight gain. No matter what people do, they cannot lose weight. They eat once a day, follow the intermittent fasting schedule, and yet they gain. Take the time to get to know a person before pointing fingers and trying to dictate to them how they should be living their lives.

Age

Illnesses, diseases, or cancers do not have a specific age target group. A six-month-old baby can be diagnosed with leukemia or a 94-year-old gentleman can be newly diagnosed with rheumatoid arthritis. Autoimmune disorders are more prevalent in women between the ages of 15 to 44. This is not to say that only certain people will be diagnosed with any one of the disorders, illnesses, or cancers.

Gut Health

Many will weigh in and say that if you have an autoimmune disorder, you are doomed and no matter what you eat or drink, your condition will not get any better. According to Amy Myers, a physician who specializes in autoimmune disorders, you need to have a healthy gut by healing your leaky gut. Your microbiome plays a major role in your overall gut health, as your digestive system is closely related to your immune system.

If you think about it, everything you eat has to go through your intestines as it is broken up and the essential nutrients are dispersed to part of your body. When you have a leaky gut, that means that the lining of your stomach has been compromised and toxins enter your system. By healing your lining, it may just be what you have been looking for and reversing any number of chronic digestive autoimmune disorders.

Gluten

Over the last couple of years, diets have been introduced whereby gluten has been the topic of heated discussions. There are those that insist that these gluten-free diets are a fad. There are others that believe that cutting gluten out of their diets is the best advice they have been given and that they have been handed a new lease on life. No two people are the same and no two people have the same conditions.

Love the idea of going gluten-free or hate it, everyone reacts differently. Some might experience bloating around the stomach area, paired with severe cramps. That would normally indicate an underlying condition. If you do find yourself suffering from gastric conditions after eating gluten products, consider getting a test for gluten intolerances. If the tests return a positive outcome, further testing for autoimmune disorders such as celiac disease would be beneficial.

Poor Quality of Life

If you are diagnosed with an autoimmune disorder, you automatically start planning your funeral. That is a fact. Everyone has had episodes where they think they have been handed a death sentence. The truth surrounding a positive diagnosis does not have to be all doom and gloom. You are in control of your life. Yes, you might have a condition that you have no control over, but you are still able to live your life to the fullest. A positive change in attitude will increase your chances of living a happy and healthy life. Every condition is manageable and sometimes all that is needed is a change here and a tweak there. Do not allow your autoimmune disorder to define who you are and what you are capable of. Make an allowance for having an off day but do not give up.

Medication

When you are first diagnosed with any illness or disease your mind tends to lead you in one direction and that would be how to cope with your particular condition. Your mind starts working and you are thinking you will not be able to cope without medication. Your doctor will prescribe medication to treat the symptoms. I am not going to tell you that, you should not be taking medication prescribed by a doctor. It is important to note that, before trying supplements or alternative medicine, to discuss these changes with your doctor. You have the right to explore all avenues, whether it be alternative therapies or supplements such as turmeric, probiotics, or omega-3 fatty acids. These are excellent supplements that help with inflammation and taking the strain off your gut lining. Other practices include meditation or yoga, which are beneficial in helping your stress and anxiety levels.

Autoimmune Disorders Reversed

With autoimmune disorders on the rise, everyone is desperate for a cure. No one wants to go through life with a debilitating illness that leaves them feeling like there is no way forward. You have been told that some of the disorders have no cures. However, some of the autoimmune disorders can be reversed by changing your habits. For these habits to be altered, you will need to look at what you are eating. Since many of the autoimmunity disorders start in the gut, it seems this is the obvious starting point. By changing your diet, stress levels, and environment, you can successfully reverse the effects of your disorder to a manageable condition.

Immune System Boost

The year the world exploded at the seams because of a global pandemic that had everyone trying everything to boost their immune systems to ensure they did not get the killer virus. Many believe that boosting their immune systems would prevent them from getting the virus, there is no substantial evidence to this statement. Matt Richtel, a journalist from the New York Times and author of the book *An Elegant Defense: The Extraordinary New Science of the Immune System* has said that "Boosting your immune system is a dangerous, ill-conceived concept and probably not even possible." (Richtel, 2019).

In an article featured in *ELLE Magazine*, Martha McCully offers various quotes relating to the immune system and what we should be doing to keep ourselves healthy. As mentioned multiple times throughout the autoimmune disorder myths, everyone agrees that ensuring you eat a healthy diet and building up your gut microbiome and lining will be a better defense mechanism in ensuring your health against viruses, bacteria, and other forms of foreign entities (McCully, 2020).

In Summary

This chapter has given you a lot of food for thought. Common misconceptions were debunked and others were reinforced. No matter what cards you are dealt, you have choices. You have been given a lot of information to know that your life is not over when you are diagnosed with an autoimmune disorder. One of the key takeaways from this chapter is that if you have any queries regarding your health status, reach out to your doctor, immunologist, or epidemiologist. Do not rely on articles or blog posts you see on the internet.

There are some catastrophic consequences to following advice from someone who thinks they know it all. Something we know which is a definite negative is not to drink bleach! You have options, and some of these options will be discussed in future chapters, but you have the right to seek second or third opinions. There are no miracle cures for autoimmune disorders. Yes, you can reverse the effects by changing your habits. You are in control. An autoimmune disorder does not have to be the end of your life. Adapt to your new life. Be hopeful that someday a cure will be found.

Chapter 4:

Autoimmune Disorders:

Types, Symptoms, and

Treatment

With everything that is happening in the world, it is understandable that we would be exposed to everything that is going around us. In saying this, no matter where in the world you are, you are exposed to an incredible amount of stress. It is easy for people to say that you should be taking time out for yourself and relaxing or meditating. When there is so much negativity and toxic energy brought on by anger, hatred, fear of the unknown, and so much more, those tiny particles latch onto a person. All these negative feelings do affect us. You may argue that nothing phases you but if you have to look deep into yourself, you will be changing your tune.

As far as our overall health is concerned, we do tend to be negligent and submissive. Everyone is focused on earning an income to put food on the table. You spend more time at the office than you do at home. It is easier to pick up the telephone or open an app on your phone to order take outs so that you can continue with your work. Has anyone ever told you that there are only 24 hours in a day? It is true. No matter how hard you try, you cannot extend those 24 hours into 30-hour days. You need time to rest. Your body needs time to heal.

A shocking reality is that autoimmune disorders are on the rise in North America. There are approximately 23.5 million Americans that have been diagnosed with having an autoimmune disorder. That is about 5% of the American population. It has previously been documented that women of childbearing years aged between 15 to 44 are at a higher risk of being diagnosed with an autoimmune disorder. Scientists at the National Institutes of Health (NIH) have done numerous studies that indicate a significant rise in the antinuclear antibodies (ANA) which is the most common biomarker in autoimmunity.

Studies

We know what autoimmunity is and we know what it is capable of doing to our bodies. We have previously mentioned that scientists are frantically researching autoimmune disorders to understand why they are wreaking havoc in our bodies. We also know that autoimmunity is when our immune system is overzealous and attacks healthy tissues, cells, and muscles. We have looked at possible factors that could contribute to these disorders. In short, we know more about what is going on than our bodies do. If they had a voice, they would let us know what is upsetting them. Technology is quite advanced but, sadly, not enough to come up with a way for our antibodies to tell us what we need to know.

Over a period of 25 years, autoimmune disorders have skyrocketed by an overwhelming 50% increase. Research continues and will continue as studies are unpacked to understand the rise in new findings. It is noted that the significant increases presented in adult males, non-Hispanic whites over the age of 50. This is a scratch the head moment to understand the surge in the autoimmune biomarker being detected in these subjects.

The studies incorporated body mass index, alcohol use, and smoking to look for answers. There are no significant explanations for the increase in ANA found in subjects. Scientists are speculating that the increase could be related to the changes in lifestyle and exposure to the ever-changing environment. It is important to note that if you have tested positive for having autoimmunity biomarkers, such as ANA, it does not mean that you have an autoimmune disorder (Dinse et al., 2020).

Different Autoimmune Disorders

Until now, you have been presented with a lot of information about what goes on inside your body. We have sidestepped drawing up your last will and testament. No one has brainwashed you into believing some outlandish theories with regards to autoimmunity. We have put some of your fears to rest. At the end of the day, you are still who you were before you arrived here.

It is crazy to imagine that there are over 90 confirmed autoimmune diseases with names. It is even crazier to think that scientists are constantly identifying more or even variants of the same disorder with different strains. We will be exploring some of the most common autoimmune disorders. Please keep in mind that this section is not about self-diagnosing symptoms you might be having. If you are displaying any type of symptoms, visit your doctor for an official diagnosis.

It is important to note that the symptoms mentioned for the various autoimmune disorders might mimic those of a typical virus such as influenza, a common cold, or gastroenteritis. If your symptoms persist or recur frequently, visit your doctor for your peace of mind. Your health is important, and your family and friends need you to stick around.

Disclaimer For the dietary inclusions presented for the various autoimmune disorders, they do not reflect the AIP diet guidelines. These mentioned have been worked out by dieticians who specialize in their various fields. It is interesting to note that there are a lot of dissimilarities when comparing the food guides. The AIP diet food lists are what you will be following.

Lupus

Lupus is an inflammatory disorder that occurs when the immune system attacks healthy tissues and organs in the body. Research has indicated that lupus is more common in women but that does not mean men and children are exempt from this chronic disorder.

Types of Lupus

Lupus is categorized into four different types. Your doctor will perform various tests which include drawing blood, urine samples, x-rays, and biopsies of inflamed tissues or organs.

- Systemic lupus erythematosus

- Cutaneous lupus

- Neonatal lupus

- Drug-induced lupus

The most common of the variants of lupus is systemic lupus erythematosus (SLE).

Symptoms

The symptoms vary from person to person. If you display any of the following symptoms, visit your doctor for a confirmed diagnosis, and to discuss your next steps.

- Aching muscles

- Shortness of breath

- Headaches

- Stiffness in the joints

- Rashes that appear for no apparent reason

- Confusion

- Loss of memory

- Unexplained bruising

- Dry and scratchy eyes

- Ulcers in the mouth

- Hair loss

- Loss of appetite

- Weight loss

Causes

No one in the medical field has come to a consensus on what causes lupus. Various factors could lead to potential triggers, but as of yet, no specific causes have been identified.

Genetics

There are more than 50 genes that have been identified by scientists that are linked to having lupus. The fact that the lupus genes have been detected in your body, does not necessarily mean you will develop the disorder. If there is a family history of lupus, there is a likelihood that you would also get it but more often than not, it does not affect everyone in the family.

Hormones

Lupus is more common in women and this could be as a result of their hormone levels. Due to a woman's menstruation cycle, they tend to produce more estrogen before they menstruate which triggers lupus symptoms. Men also produce estrogen but on a lighter scale, which is why more women than men are diagnosed with lupus.

Environment

We can play the blame game and point fingers at everything around us that might be potential triggers for being diagnosed with diseases or disorders. Some of the most common triggers that stand out when analyzing lupus is being exposed to cigarette smoke or smoking, stress, or inhaling toxins, such as silica dust, as well as certain viruses.

Risk Factors

In addition to the causes mentioned, several risk factors can contribute to the theory of being diagnosed with lupus.

Gender

As previously mentioned, women are at a greater risk of a lupus diagnosis than men.

Age

Most sufferers are diagnosed between the ages of 15 to 44. These ages are in no way set in stone and anyone of any age can be diagnosed.

Ethnicity

It is believed that African Americans, Native Americans, and Hispanics are at a greater risk of being diagnosed with lupus, it is not to say that it is only limited to a specific group.

Treatment

Scientists and researchers have yet to find a cure for this chronic disorder. There are various options available to help treat the symptoms and manage any pain or discomfort you might be experiencing. In some instances, due to the severe pain, medication is administered to treat swelling, inflammation, protect your organs from severe damage, and tame the immune system.

A holistic approach to managing pain and discomfort include:

- Stop smoking

- Vitamin D

- Calcium

- Fish oil

- Exercise

- Avoiding unnecessary exposure to ultraviolet light

Overview

We know that there is no cure for lupus and it is something you will have to live with for the rest of your life. There may be days, weeks, or months that go by without any indication that you have lupus. Many will think that they have been cured until any number of triggers remind them that all is not well. Regardless of the severity of your condition, you are, will, and can live a normal life. Do not be complacent when it comes to your treatment. If you suspect a new symptom, seek medical help for confirmation.

Rheumatoid Arthritis (RA)

Rheumatoid Arthritis is an inflammatory disorder that affects the joints in your body. The condition is however not limited to the joints but can affect the skin, lungs, head, eyes, and blood vessels.

Types of rheumatoid arthritis

There are various types of rheumatoid arthritis, with seropositive RA being the most common affecting more than 1.3 million Americans. RA is diagnosed after a blood test is positive for a protein marker called rheumatoid factor or an antibody named anti-cyclic citrullinated peptide.

- Seropositive RA

- Seronegative RA

- Juvenile idiopathic arthritis

Symptoms

- Waking up with stiff joints

- Constantly tired, even after a seemingly good night's rest

- Joint pains

- Swelling in the region of joints

- Fever

- Tingles throughout your body

- Loss of feeling

- Struggling to sleep

- Lack of appetite

- Weight loss

Causes and Risk Factors

As with all autoimmune disorders, there are no specific causes as to why your immune system would attack healthy tissues or organs. There are various factors that may play a role leading to your diagnosis. Various genes might contribute to the diagnosis of RA, but a battery of blood tests will offer confirmation.

Genetics

It is believed that if there is a history of RA in your family, that you could be at risk of being diagnosed.

Age

Depending on which strain of RA you are diagnosed with, you could develop symptoms as early as three years of age (JIA). There is no specific age group or timeline when you can develop RA.

Gender

Again, women are at a higher risk of developing RA. Men are not to be too complacent with this news, as they too can be diagnosed.

Environment

Although there is no concrete evidence that environmental issues are to blame for RA, it is believed that being exposed to asbestos or silica dust may be a trigger.

Lifestyle

Smokers are admonished to give up their smelly habit, as this increases your genetic markers to develop RA. Obesity is believed to be a trigger for RA as when you are carrying around extra weight, you are putting unnecessary strain on your joints and ligaments which will cause inflammation.

Treatment

While there are no cures for RA, there are various treatments and holistic approaches to coping with the pain and discomfort. It is always best to speak to your doctor about your intentions of using home remedies. Nine times out of 10, your doctor will give you the green light.

Home remedies that might alleviate pain and discomfort include:

- Low impact exercise such as yoga

- Rest

- Hot or cold compresses to the affected areas or warm showers to ease the stiffness you might be experiencing.

- Braces, crutches, or canes

Overview

There is no cure for rheumatoid arthritis. You will encounter days where you have pain that feels as if your body is burning from the inside or you might feel as if your joints are about to snap off. With the correct treatment, a healthy diet free of inflammatory-inducing foods, and some home remedies, you can live a long and fulfilling life. If the pain and discomfort become unbearable, contact your doctor or go in for a consultation.

Type 1 Diabetes

Type 1 diabetes is an autoimmune disorder where the antibodies attack the beta cells in the pancreas. The pancreas is a vital organ that produces insulin which regulates your blood sugar. According to the American Diabetes Association, there are approximately 1.25 million Americans that suffer from type 1 diabetes.

Types

Type 1 diabetes is not to be confused with type 2 diabetes. Type 1 diabetes deals with the production of insulin, type 2 diabetes patients do not respond to the insulin that is being produced making them insulin resistant.

Symptoms

Diabetes is not a disease that should be taken lightly. If you experience any of the following symptoms, it is strongly advised to visit your doctor for a diagnosis. Patients with type 1 diabetes can develop complications which are known as ketoacidosis.

Normal symptoms include:

- Blurry vision

- Exhaustion

- Constantly thirsty

- Constantly hungry

- Urinating more frequently

- Excessive weight loss

Ketoacidosis symptoms include:

- Dry skin

- Pasty mouth

- Rapid breathing

- Constantly nauseous

- Stomach cramps

- Vomiting

- A sweet or fruity-smelling breath

Risk Factors

There are no specific causes as to why the body would be attacking the beta cells but scientists have noted that there are some risk factors that could contribute to the eventual diagnosis.

Genetics

It is believed that a history of diabetes in the family could increase the chances of someone being diagnosed. Type 1 diabetes is a rare disorder but early detection is the key to efficiently managing the condition.

Age

Diabetes does not have a specific timeline for when you can show symptoms or be potentially diagnosed. Patients with type 1 diabetes are diagnosed by the time they turn 30. That being said, you are never too old or too young to be diagnosed.

Treatment

Modern medicine intervention is required for the treatment of type 1 diabetes. Patients need to monitor their blood sugar levels multiple times a day. Levels are recorded by a simple finger prick and then administering insulin. There are two ways in which patients can replenish their insulin which is either through injections or an insulin pump. Some might not be too comfortable with sticking a needle in their bodies, so a pump is a better option. Thanks to modern technology, insulin pumps are triggered to detect an increase or drop in blood sugar levels. Due to constant research, new medications are being developed that could possibly replace injections and pumps.

It should also be noted that patients with type 1 diabetes should be eating regularly to keep the blood sugar levels on an even keel. Exercise also plays a role in keeping blood sugar levels at a comfortable level.

Overview

There are no known cures for type 1 diabetes but following the treatment action plan, there are no reasons not to live a healthy life. Lifestyle changes such as a healthy diet and limiting or even eliminating alcohol, are beneficial to manage your condition.

Thyroid Diseases

The thyroid gland is found at the base of the neck and is important to your body as it controls your metabolism. Having a well-functioning metabolism is vital to the overall health and well-being of a person. The thyroid forms part of a network of glands known as the endocrine system which produces chemicals and hormones that keep the body working. The thyroid hormones play an important role in our bodies as it regulates body functions. We will be exploring Grave's disease and Hashimoto's thyroiditis in the next section.

Grave's Disease

Grave's disease is commonly known as hyperthyroidism. It is believed to be the most common thyroid disorder. Antibodies connect with healthy cells and the thyroid gland starts producing too many hormones for the body to process.

Symptoms

- Weight loss

- Increased heart rate

- Shaking hands

- Weakened muscles

- Insomnia

- Swollen glands in the neck

- Exhaustion

- Irritation

- Anxiousness or nervous

If you display any of the symptoms listed, you can visit your doctor for confirmation. Your doctor will perform various tests to confirm your diagnosis.

Causes and Risk Factors

There are no specific causes as to why the antibodies attack healthy thyroid cells. Scientists have identified some risks that could lead to a positive diagnosis.

Genetics

A history of Grave's disease in the family could increase the chances of being diagnosed. Should you have the Grave's genes in your body, it is not to say that you will be diagnosed.

Gender

Although not gender-specific, it is believed that women are more susceptible to a positive diagnosis.

Age

Patients are usually diagnosed before the age of 40.

Conditions

Pre-existing autoimmune disorders such as type 1 diabetes and/or rheumatoid arthritis increase the likelihood of a positive diagnosis for Grave's disease.

Lifestyle

Stress and smoking are believed to be trigger agents for people who have the Grave's genes. It is strongly recommended that smokers consider changing their habits to avoid complications associated with Grave's disease such as Grave's ophthalmopathy.

Treatment

- Anti-thyroid medication

- Surgery

- Radioactive iodine therapy

Overview

As of yet, there are no known cures for Grave's disease. There are various treatments available. There is no known reason or cause to believe that someone who is diagnosed with Grave's disease cannot live a long and happy life.

Hashimoto's Thyroiditis

Hashimoto's Thyroiditis is known as hypothyroidism. We previously learned that hyperthyroidism occurs when the antibodies create too many hormones which speed up the metabolism. In contrast, hyperthyroidism occurs when the antibodies prevent the thyroid gland from producing the much-needed hormones that are necessary to keep our energy levels up. The most noticeable symptom of an under-active thyroid is unexplained weight gain. Many of the symptoms mimic those of Grave's disease.

Symptoms

- Constipation

- Hoarseness when speaking

- Depression

- Exhaustion

- Lethargy

- Constantly cold

- Irregular menstruation cycle

- Cholesterol

- Weakness to the lower part of the body

- Pale skin color

- Fertility issues

Risk Factors

While there are no specific causes as to what causes Hashimoto's thyroiditis, there are various risk factors that can be identified.

Genetics

If anyone in your direct family has been diagnosed with Hashimoto's, it would be advisable to have tests done to confirm. It is believed that if someone in your family has been diagnosed, the chances of a positive diagnosis are greater.

Gender

Hashimoto's is not a gender-specific disorder but the majority of patients that are diagnosed are women.

Age

Anyone of any age can be diagnosed but the majority of patients are diagnosed in their middle-aged years.

Conditions

Pre-existing autoimmune disorders such as rheumatoid arthritis, type 1 diabetes, and/or lupus are believed to increase the likelihood of a positive diagnosis.

Environment

Exposure to higher than normal levels of radiation could increase the possibility of being diagnosed with Hashimoto's.

Treatment

There are various supplements and medications that can be used to control the condition. It is important to consult your doctor before taking any medication or supplements. Your doctor will be able to work out an efficient treatment plan.

Possible supplements and medication would include:

- Hormone therapy

- Cholesterol medication

- Calcium

- Iron

- Acid reflux medication

Overview

Do not ignore the symptoms mentioned. Symptoms might seem generic and recur more often than not, it could be a sign of an underlying condition. For your peace of mind, consult your doctor. There are various complications that could occur if you let you ignore the symptoms. Remember, your family and friends need you.

Psoriasis

Psoriasis is a skin condition that occurs when the T cells in your body mistakenly attack the skin cells causing a rapid buildup of skin. As the new skin is being produced and forced out to make way for more skin, the old skin cells do not know how to cope with the regeneration and it continues to build up.

Symptoms

Psoriasis can be found on elbows, the scalp, legs, or in rare cases, in the groin area.

- White to silver flakes

- Itching

- Pain around the target area/s

- Dry skin

- Red patches on the skin

- Warm to hot to the touch

No two people have the same symptoms. If you suspect you have a skin condition, visit your doctor for a definitive diagnosis. Your doctor will perform a physical examination to examine the areas of concern. If further confirmation is needed, you will be sent for a biopsy where laboratory technicians will analyze the skin sample.

Causes and Risk Factors

There are no known causes for the onset of psoriasis other than the explanation of the T cells attacking the skin producing cells in the body. There are however risk factors and triggers which could lead to a confirmed diagnosis.

Genetics

Psoriasis is a condition that is passed on through the bloodline. The possibility of an offspring developing the condition is high, and even higher if both parents have the same condition. This is not to say that it is limited to families, as anyone can be diagnosed at some point in their lives.

Lifestyle

Lifestyle plays a huge part in triggering psoriasis in someone who has the gene. A lifestyle change, before the onset of symptoms and consequently a diagnosis, would be advised.

- Reduce stress

- Stop smoking

- Limit alcohol consumption

Environment

The weather is a factor that cannot be reckoned with. Psoriasis does not like cold, dry weather conditions.

Treatment

There are no known cures for psoriasis and treatments include medications, moisturizer, and light therapy. There are a couple of lifestyle changes that can help to manage the pain and discomfort experienced.

Diet

It is recommended that the use of saturated fats found in animal products be limited. Focus on eating lean cuts of protein that are high in omega-3 fatty acids, as well as walnuts, soybeans, and flaxseed. Avoid or limit red meat, processed food, dairy, and refined sugar.

Overview

Being diagnosed and living with psoriasis is not the end of the world. If taken care of and making use of the recommendations and advice given, you can manage your condition. Keep your skin hydrated by making use of moisturizer or unperfumed lotions. Do not pick off your flakes, as you might scratch a patch of skin and cause an infection.

Psoriatic Arthritis

Psoriatic Arthritis is an autoimmune disorder that affects patients with psoriasis. Arthritis is a condition that mimics rheumatoid arthritis affecting joints. There are various types of psoriatic arthritis that affect various parts of the body such as the hands and feet, the joints close to the nails, or the spine.

Symptoms

- Stiff joints in the morning

- Swelling on either or both sides of the body

- Aching muscles

- Flaky skin and/or scalp

- Red eyes

- Pain in the eyes

- Exhaustion

The severe psoriatic arthritis condition that affects the spine, spondylitis PsA, presents symptoms of pain, weakness, and/or swelling of:

- Spine

- Toes

- Fingers

- Feet

- Ankles

- Wrists

- Elbows

Risk Factors

There are risk factors that could determine the diagnosis of psoriatic arthritis.

Psoriasis

Having this pre-existing condition increases the risk of developing psoriatic arthritis.

Genetics

Family members such as parents and offspring are at risk of adding arthritis to their existing condition.

Age

There is no age limit as to when psoriatic arthritis can develop but the average age is between 30 to 50 years.

Lifestyle Changes

As with most conditions and disorders, a simple lifestyle change could help with maintaining your condition and keeping you comfortable.

- Stop smoking

- Limit alcohol consumption

- Avoid unnecessary stress

- Keep moving to keep your joints and muscles supple

- Diet

- Incorporate anti-inflammatory foods such as omega-3 fatty acids

- Spices such as turmeric

- Eat a well-balanced diet

- Eat more fresh fruits

- Eat more fresh vegetables

- Limit the consumption of processed foods

Treatment

There are no cures available. Your doctor will prescribe a plan of action consisting of medication that is to be used per the treatment plan.

Multiple Sclerosis (MS)

Multiple Sclerosis is an incurable disorder where antibodies attack the nerves in the central nervous system. These attacks cause scarring on the tissues, inflammation, and/or lesions. The damage caused makes it difficult for the brain to send functional signals to the body.

Symptoms

Patients with MS are faced with many symptoms that seem to appear overnight or over a period of time.

- Exhaustion

- Weak muscles

- Numb feet or hands

- Off-balance

- Blurry vision

- Slurring speech

- Concentration

- Muscle spasms

- Severe pain

If you experience any of these symptoms, visit your doctor who will perform various tests to diagnose your condition. These tests could include blood samples, MRI scans, eye exams, or a lumbar puncture.

Risk Factors

There are various risk factors that could play a role in the development of MS.

Genetics

If parents or siblings are diagnosed with MS, the chances of a positive diagnosis are high.

Age

MS is not age-specific and can affect people of all ages.

Gender

The majority of patients being diagnosed with MS are women.

Ethnicity

It is believed that white people pose a higher risk of being diagnosed with MS.

Conditions

Pre-existing conditions such as thyroid disease, type 1 diabetes, inflammatory bowel disease, or psoriasis wave a high-risk flag of warning for possibly being diagnosed with MS.

Treatment

There are no known cures for MS but there are various medications that your doctor will incorporate into your treatment action plan. While there might not be a cure for MS, a holistic approach could be incorporated into your new way of life. Before you make any changes to your lifestyle, consult your doctor, and clue him/her in on your intentions.

Diet

Eat a well-balanced diet that is high in fiber and essential nutrients. Consider eliminating or limiting the consumption of processed food, saturated and trans fats, sugar drinks and foods, and high-sodium products.

Exercise

Keeping the muscles and joints supple require some work from the host. As difficult as it may be to even get out of bed in the morning, keep moving. Practice yoga, go for short walks, participate in water aerobics at the gym, or swim in your neighbor's pool.

Inflammatory Bowel Disease (IBD)

Inflammatory bowel disease is a collective name for different types of disorders that affect the intestines. These disorders originate in the digestive tract which is made up of the mouth, stomach, small intestine, large intestine, and esophagus. The digestive tract is responsible for breaking down the food and sending it to the appropriate parts of the body.

Types

Two common disorders stem from inflammatory bowel disease which we will be taking a closer look further in this chapter.

Crohn's Disease

The digestive tract is susceptible to inflammation caused by Chron's disease. The small intestine is more vulnerable to inflammatory reactions.

Ulcerative Colitis

The large intestine becomes inflamed.

Symptoms

- Stomach pain

- Stomach cramps

- Distended stomach

- Bleeding ulcers

- Diarrhea

- Weight loss

- Anemia

- Inflammation of the eyes

- Skin conditions

- Joint conditions

Diagnosis

If you have any of the symptoms mentioned here, visit your doctor who will perform tests to confirm your condition as well as define which of the two disorders you have possibly developed.

Crohn's Disease

As we have learned, there are two types of inflammatory bowel disease that are placed under one umbrella. Each of these disorders affects a different part of the intestine. Crohn's disease presents in the small intestine. While not limited to the small intestine, it can affect the colon as well as the digestive tract that leads from the mouth to the anus.

Symptoms

- Stomach cramps

- Bloody stools

- Diarrhea

- Fever

- Exhaustion

- No appetite

- Weight loss

- A feeling of fullness in your bowel is going to the toilet

These symptoms mimic the regular stomach ailments after eating too much, a stomach virus, or food poisoning. If your symptoms recur or do not let up, visit your doctor for a checkup. If left untreated or not diagnosed properly, your symptoms could become worse.

- Unexplained ulcers

- Skin and joints become inflamed

- An onset of shortness of breath when doing anything physical such as walk to a room

Risk Factors

Genetics

Your chances of developing Crohn's disease are significantly higher if a close blood relative such as a parent or offspring has been diagnosed.

Age

There is no specific age category for developing Crohn's disease but it is believed that most patients are diagnosed before the age of 30.

Ethnicity

This disease does not choose you based on your race and it can develop in anyone. There has been mention of Crohn's disease showing an increase in the African American community.

Lifestyle

Patients with Crohn's disease are told that smoking is to be stopped with immediate effect. Smoking leads to severe symptoms as well as the need for surgery.

Treatment

Once diagnosed, your doctor will work out a treatment plan and prescribe anti-inflammatory medication and/or antibiotics. You can also help your body by making some dietary changes. Certain food causes your intestines to react negatively and leave you in more pain than is necessary. In some instances, depending on the severity of your condition, surgery is the only option to remove the damaged part of your intestine and reconnect it to the healthy part.

Dietary Changes

While there are no cures for Crohn's disease, you can implement some changes to help keep your intestines happy. Keep a food diary of what you eat and note any side effects of eating certain foods. Some of the areas to adjust to your diet are as follows:

- Fiber

- Fats

- Dairy

- Drink more water

Ulcerative Colitis

The second of the two types of inflammatory bowel diseases is called ulcerative colitis. Where Crohn's disease affects the digestive tract from the mouth to the anus along the small intestine, ulcerative colitis affects the large intestine or colon. The lining of the large intestine and/or the rectum is inflamed. When inflammation occurs, ulcers are formed along the lining of the large intestine starting at the rectum and spreading. This will result in the frequency of emptying your bowels. If left untreated, the ulcers could result in bleeding and mucus and/or pus discharge.

Symptoms

- Stomach cramps

- Sounds coming from your stomach

- Diarrhea

- Fever

- Blood in the stools

- Weight loss

- Malnutrition

- Pain in the joints

- Swelling around the joints

- Nausea

- Loss of appetite

- Skin conditions

- Ulcers

- Inflammation of the eyes

Risk Factors

Genetics

If you have a close relative that has ulcerative colitis, you are at risk of developing this disorder.

Age

There is no specific age category to develop ulcerative colitis. Most people are diagnosed before the age of 30 but also presents in patients after they turn 60.

Ethnicity

White people have a higher risk of developing ulcerative colitis but it can affect all races.

Treatment

Your doctor will work out a treatment plan and prescribe medication. Depending on the severity of the condition, surgery would be needed. Surgery would be the removal of the colon or part thereof. This is a worst-case scenario. This surgery is called a colostomy where a pathway is created through the lining of your stomach to the surface. You will then be fitted with a bag for your waste to go into a special bag that has to be cleaned out multiple times a day.

Dietary Changes

In order to avoid surgery, it would be strongly advised to change your diet. This is not meant to be a scare tactic, but it could be a reality if you do not take care of yourself.

- Consume a low-fat diet

- Increase your vitamin C intake

- Increase your healthy fiber

Celiac Disease

Celiac Disease is a chronic disorder that affects your digestive system. This disorder occurs when your immune system has a negative reaction to gluten. Our small intestines consist of villi which mimic small fingers along the lining. The purpose of the villi is to absorb nutrients from the food we consume. In celiac disease, when you consume gluten, your immune system creates harmful toxins that damage or destroy the villi.

Symptoms

The symptoms of celiac disease are different for adults and children.

Children

- Tiredness
- Irritable/cranky
- Vomiting
- Constipated
- Runny stools
- Pale stools
- Fatty stools
- Stomach cramps
- Bloating

Adults

- Anemia, which is a sign of iron deficiency

- Exhaustion

- Skin conditions

- Joint pain

- Stiffness in the joints

- Seizures

- Pins and needles sensation in the hands and feet

- Discolored teeth

- Mouth sores

- Weak/brittle bones

- Infertility

- Miscarriage

- Irregular menstrual cycle

Some people might have been diagnosed with celiac disease but have had no symptoms. This does not mean they have been cured and can eat gluten again. Treat your symptom-free diagnosis as if you have symptoms. Do not compare your symptoms with others who have the same disorder. There are a couple of factors that make it difficult to compare one case to another.

- Length of time being breastfed

- Age when being introduced to gluten products

- Amount of gluten being consumed

- How badly the intestines have been damaged

If you suspect you have celiac disease, visit your doctor for an official diagnosis as soon as possible.

Risk Factors

Genetics

If you have a family member that has celiac disease, the chance of a positive diagnosis is high.

Diagnosed Disorders

If you have any of the following disorders, the possibility of being diagnosed with celiac disease is high.

- Rheumatoid arthritis

- Lupus

- Thyroid disease

- Addison's disease

- Colon cancer

- Lymphoma of the colon

- Intolerant to lactose

- Autoimmune hepatitis

Diagnosing

Diagnosing celiac disease will involve a physical and exploring your family and medical history. Further testing will include full blood work looking at how the liver functions and cholesterol levels.

Treatment

Until a confirmed diagnosis has been determined, patients should refrain from consuming anything gluten related.

Items to Avoid

- Semolina

- Wheat

- Rye

- Barley

- Graham flour

- Durum

- Candy

- Cakes

- Beer

- Cookies

- Pies

- Cereals

- Croutons

- Oats

- Pasta

- Processed meat

- Salad dressing

Items to Include

- Fresh meat

- Fruit

- Dairy

- Vegetables

In Summary

When you look at the statistics saying that 23.5 million North Americans have been diagnosed with autoimmune disorders, you have started wondering how you can prevent this from happening. Start with yourself. Be an advocate for your body and retrain your body by making conscious choices. You got a sneak peek at some of the autoimmune disorders. You saw the risk factors. You saw dietary recommendations.

These disorders we looked at are a drop in the ocean. There are many more that we have not mentioned but there are disorders that affect every part of our bodies. To date, there are no cures. Will food help cure your disorder? No, but it will help keep your condition under control. All it will take is a little bit of effort from you, mixed with tears of frustration. Do not lose hope.

Chapter 5:

Can Nutrition Really Help?

If you have done independent research about your particular disorder, you have been given all kinds of advice from well-meaning family members, friends, or strangers. One of the most frequent pieces of advice that you have been presented with while reading about the various risk factors leading to autoimmune disorders is to stop smoking. The second most frequent is changing your diet. You open a magazine and you see advertisements about how following a certain diet has helped cure some or other disorder. You see advertisements while watching YouTube videos telling you that your disorder is curable and if you click on the link provided, you will get more information. All these advertisements do is offer false hope and end up costing you a fortune as you have to purchase a whole shopping cart full of supplements and whatnot.

Can nutrition really help? Can changing your diet really cure a chronic autoimmune disorder? That is the million-dollar question. We have established that there is no scientific evidence leading up to believe that there are cures for these disorders. This does not mean that a cure will never be developed. Scientists are hard at work researching autoimmune disorders, but as of yet, there has been no conclusive evidence of any cures. In addition to searching for cures, scientists have been researching the relationship between autoimmune disorders and food. Maybe one day, in the not too distant future, someone will find a cure to all 90 plus autoimmune diseases. We are allowed to live in hope.

Food Versus Medication

You often hear advice from people about how you should incorporate a certain food, herb, or spice into your diet to combat a certain illness or disorder. There are testimonies from people who have suffered from a disorder and that by eating more of this and less than that, their disorder was miraculously cured. This revelation sends everyone running to the store or farmer's market to mass purchase this miracle cure. We have established that there are no known cures for autoimmune disorders. That is the reality and people are so desperate, they will believe in anything to help them, regardless of the consequences. I do not want to give anyone false hope.

We are living in a world that is constantly changing. New foods are introduced, new medications are developed and more people are diagnosed with any number of illnesses, disorders, or cancer. The whole world is up in arms and this is where the sofa doctors have weighed in with their "medical expertise." Eat more of this and less of that, stop doing this and do more of that, or drink this and not that. We are adults. We know the consequences of our habits. There comes a time when we throw our arms up and declare defeat, rush out to the closest fast-food restaurant, or dive into a double fudge brownie. What works for one person will not necessarily work for another. Deep down, we know that we need to implement positive changes to our lifestyles, especially focusing on our nutrition.

No one is going to tell you to stop taking your prescription medication. You have been prescribed your medication for a purpose. If you do experience a change by altering your diet, speak to your doctor. Get an official confirmation but do not stop until you have had a thorough checkup.

Dietary Modification

You have more control over your health than you give yourself credit for. You have the ability to make conscious decisions. You are here because you are looking for a way to manage your disorder/s. That was a conscious decision you made to help yourself. That is a massive step that deserves a pat on the back.

Health Food

Vitamins and minerals are beneficial to our overall health. You might be frowning and saying that you take supplements. There is nothing wrong with taking supplements. A nutritious meal will offer a variety of essential vitamins and minerals that are vital to your body. It is also worth mentioning that our bodies don't need copious amounts of vitamins to perform its purpose. Whatever your body does not absorb will be passed through your system.

Plant Foods

Our bodies need to produce antioxidants which are important in assisting the antibodies to fight harmful pathogens. Eating nutritious whole foods such as fruit, vegetables, and grains helps produce antioxidants that will protect lymphocyte cells from harm.

Fiber

Fiber is something everyone needs to keep the digestive system operating. It is also important for keeping your gut microbiome happy and healthy. Eating foods high in fiber can help with inflammation, as well as strengthen the immune system.

Amino Acids

Amino acids are found in protein. If you are vegan or vegetarian, I am not about to tell you that you need to eat animal products. Our bodies do not produce the amino acids we need to fulfill the essential role our immune systems need to function. By incorporating protein such as meat, poultry, dairy, eggs, seafood, quinoa, buckwheat, and soy into our diets, we are helping our immune system, strengthening our muscles, and regulating our metabolisms.

Fats

Yes, fats are a vital additive to our diets. No, do not think about slathering your toast with a thick layer of butter. When we talk about fats, we are talking about omega-3 fats. Foods rich in omega-3 fats include salmon, sardines, walnuts, chia seeds, flax seeds, anchovies, and cod liver oil. Vegetables such as spinach and Brussel sprouts could be incorporated into your diet as they contain small amounts of omega-3 fats.

Good versus Bad

There is no time like the present to start implementing a change to your lifestyle. Since the beginning of 2020, most of us have been sitting at home baking banana bread, sourdough bread, muffins, and not caring about what we put into our bodies. We have been living the quarantine life where we were prohibited from going to work, visiting friends and family, and not exercising at the gym. Many might disagree with this assumption but the reality is, limitations were put in place and we had to adapt to our new normal.

We need to hold ourselves accountable for the choices we make when it comes to what we put into our bodies. Unhealthy choices lead to consequences such as health issues leading to a wide range of diseases and disorders. Change can be overwhelming but with perseverance, anything can be achieved. Your health is important and your family needs you to stick around for as long as possible.

Switch out the unhealthy foods and replace them with healthier nutritious options. No one is telling you that you should never eat a piece of candy or a cookie. If you want it, have one but in moderation. If you want a hamburger, fries, and milkshake from your favorite fast-food restaurant, consider putting your meal together from scratch. For every unhealthy food option, you have the resources to make your own and you have control over what you add. Convenience food saves time but at what cost to our health?

Gut Health

By now we know that everything we put in our mouth has to go somewhere. There is a whole factory inside our body that, whether we want to admit it or not, we take for granted. This factory is known as your microbiome. Our microbiome consists of microbes which collectively make up a community of healthy bacteria, viruses, and fungi. As we previously mentioned, our immune systems are special to us. The same can be said for the microbes. In the same way that our antibodies are trained to keep us healthy, the microbes have a pretty difficult job to do by working hard to ensure our guts are working like well-oiled machines.

This might seem a little daunting, considering I mentioned that you have bugs, viruses, bacteria, and fungi living in your gut. Your microbiome acts in the same way as your immune system does, except it does not create antibodies to ward off diseases and infections. When you eat something, that item of food has to work its way down, around, and through the digestive tract. Your microbiome is responsible for breaking down the food, separating the good from the bad, and compartmentalizing everything. Once the process has been completed, the waste works itself out of the body, and the nutrients are sent to the appropriate organs, tissues, muscles, and joints to face the immune system.

Remember, nothing is perfect and issues do occur. Our bodies are no exception. As with the immune system and the battle of good versus good, our microbiomes have a similar issue. Something will slip through the factory that wasn't broken down and identified. The pathogen will make its way through the intestines and leave a trail of destruction in its wake. Potential health issues could develop ranging from 24-hour bugs to more severe ailments. The bottom line is, the microbiome is defined by the food we eat. If we do not take care of our microbiome, we could be pathing the way for a whole host of issues such as weight gain or long-term disorders.

Leaky Gut Syndrome

Many doctors are on the fence about whether the leaky gut syndrome is a real medical condition. Scientists have come up with evidence which they hope would sway the medical profession to recognize the signs. When we mention the gut, we know it has something to do with our stomachs and intestines. We have an understanding of how the food that enters our bodies are processed. Our intestines act as a barrier and help the food move along to where it needs to go. As much as we are not perfect, our intestines also have their 'off' moments and problems arise.

The barrier walls of our intestines are compromised for whatever reason. Cracks appear and before our food is broken down properly, unidentified bacteria or toxins break through the barrier and enter our bloodstream. These harmful pathogens trigger the immune system into producing antibodies which could ultimately lead to identifying the wrong enemies and confusing the antibodies into fighting healthy cells.

Symptoms

- Sensitive to certain foods

- Skin conditions

- Excessive gas

- Swelling or bloating around the stomach area

- Exhaustion

- Problems digesting food

Risk Factors

While not written in stone, these risk factors are likely to play a role in the way your gut reacts.

- Alcohol Consumption

- Use of certain medications

- Sugar

- Stress

- Gut health

- Not getting the correct nutrients

- Too much yeast being produced

Possible Disorders

Remembering that the medical profession is still on the wall about acknowledging that leaky gut syndrome is a real medical condition, various disorders have been linked.

- Celiac disease

- Crohn's disease

- Diabetes

- Food allergies

- Irritable Bowel Syndrome

There are many disorders and illnesses that are claimed to be directly related to leaky gut syndrome but the evidence is sparse or unfounded.

Improving Gut Health

- Gut healthy fermented foods free of additives

- Fiber-enriched foods

- Probiotics

- Limit carbohydrates that are refined

- Limit over-the-counter medication

You Are What You Eat

This is a statement we have seen or heard so many times that it makes you feel self-conscious. You end up eating in secret and avoid eating at dinner parties or restaurants. People are ruthless in the way they judge a person based on their outward appearance. You can see the disgust on their faces when they see you eating something that is probably not on the healthy spectrum. People are quick to judge without really understanding what the other person might be going through.

According to research conducted by a group of scientists in 2014, what you eat makes a difference in how the immune system responds. Considering that the food you consume gets broken down by your microbiome, some foods and additives are harder to break down due to their compositions. It is believed that the westernized diet, which consists of large amounts of saturated fats, sucrose, and less fiber, is responsible for many of our health and dietary problems we are faced with. One of the biggest concerns with the westernized diet is that it leads to obesity. The yo-yo effect comes into play as obesity is linked to many types of autoimmune disorders such as thyroid disease, diabetes, hypertension, or inflammation (Manzel, et al, 2014).

Something we have mentioned numerous times is that no two people are the same. No two people's bodies work the same way. Some people are just blessed to have a body that can tolerate more while others struggle. Some have to work harder than others. We cannot point fingers and sneer at those who have a different body type because, in a year or three, the roles could be reversed.

An Untold Story

During my research, I came across a middle-aged lady who was severely obese. I was horrified. She presented as a ticking time bomb for all kinds of illnesses and disorders. I started asking questions and she looked me in the eye and answered without looking away. The more she spoke, the more I changed my opinion. For the purpose of telling her story, we will call her Marge.

Marge grew up in a loving home with her parents. She was an only child until the age of 10. Marge had always been a 'big' child but all that changed when her sibling was born. The attention Marge had been getting had shifted to the new baby. Grandparents and family did not acknowledge her and seemed to push her aside. Marge looked for attention in the pantry. Over the years, as her sibling got older, the bullying started. The sibling knew which buttons to press to get attention, and since Marge was never an attention seeker, she withdrew into herself and found solace in her snacks, especially crisps and salty foods.

By the time Marge was 16, she was so overweight that she needed special school clothing. She endured a lot of name-calling and bullying from her schoolmates but she put on a brave smile each day and even laughed with them. Her parents tried their best to help her. They put her on diets. They took her to doctors. They tried everything but Marge could not lose weight. At this point, Marge had stopped eating junk foods and was basically eating lean meat, vegetables without butter, and salads. Her aunt and cousins embarrassed her at every chance they could by making her try on their clothes and jeering at her when their skinny clothes couldn't move over her hips.

Marge had built up a brick wall around herself and avoided going to family gatherings. She had never told her parents about what the family was doing. A huge sigh of relief for Marge was when her family was relocated to another state. Just the relief of knowing that she would not be seeing them frequently started a transformation and Marge started losing weight. The weight loss was short-lived because the sibling started taunting her. It was a vicious circle.

Fast forward about 15 years, Marge had a health scare. She developed an abscess in her breast. No matter how she tried to ignore the excruciating pain, inflammation, and swelling, she was rushed to the emergency room. The doctors were baffled and started prodding and eventually before a biopsy could be done, they had said that it was breast cancer. I have to mention here, that all the doctor's Marge had seen as a teenager, had given her a clean bill of health. There were no signs of diabetes, thyroid disease, cholesterol, or hypertension. At the appointment to find out the fate of her biopsy, her doctor told her that it was definitely not cancer.

The doctor asked some questions, felt around, and did a few more tests. It was eventually discovered that Marge had a tear in her stomach lining. They suspected a hernia and possibly inflammatory bowel disease due to a family history of colon cancer. It was further discovered that Marge had the leaky gut syndrome. The pieces of the puzzle started to fit together. It took 40 years for them to make this discovery. Marge is on her way to reclaiming her health by having changed her diet. One of the main culprits is carbohydrates, especially processed carbohydrates such as bread, sugar, rice, and pasta. Marge is slowly adjusting to her new way of life. She says it is not easy and every day is a battle. She showed me some photos of her progress and my mouth hung open.

Instead of judging someone by the way they look, put yourself in their shoes. Every person is unique. Every person has a story. Marge walked around for 40 years before being diagnosed. She is doing the best she can given her circumstances. Marge, we wish you well and look forward to the day that you appear in the news with your story.

In Summary

Can nutrition really help? We know that there are no cures for autoimmune disorders. By implementing some nutritional practices, you will be able to manage your disorder. Do not stand back and accept your disorder as being a death sentence. Start implementing some of the changes today. Where you took two teaspoons of sugar in your coffee, take one and steadily cut down until you do not need that sweetness. Where you were eating fast-food five times a week, skip a day or two, and start preparing your meals yourself. Before you know it, you do not need that fast-food because your homemade meals taste much better. A bonus is that you will be saving money. Okay, money has nothing to do with our immune systems but it is nice to know that by saving money, you are not worrying about finances which cause undue stress.

Anything is possible when you put your mind to it. Your health and well-being are important. You are tired of the pain and discomfort you are experiencing. What have you got to lose by changing what you eat?

Chapter 6:

Join Forces With the

Autoimmune Protocol Diet

How wonderful life would be if everyone could eat and drink whatever they wanted without worrying about what would happen to their bodies? Everyone has tried some or other diet in their lifetime, whether they care to admit it or not. It seems that a lot of people are afraid to admit that they are following a program to help them lose weight, gain weight, build muscle, or for the health benefits they offer. No matter what diet or lifestyle we are following, our actions will be scrutinized. We live in a cruel world where our perfect imperfections are pointed out by those who need to take stock of their situations. No one should ever be made to feel embarrassed about the way they look.

The market is saturated with different diets and lifestyles that claim to be the answer to your prayers or the secret to shedding a couple of pounds with little effort. Everyone will have an opinion about which diet is THE best. Not every diet will have the same effect on people, and results may differ. Weighing up the pros and the cons, ticking the relevant boxes that apply, and making a list with your health concerns in mind might be trickier than imagined. Each diet offers its own reasoning as to why it would be beneficial.

We both know why you are here. The title of this book is a dead giveaway. Maybe you have done some independent research and are trying to get answers about how to deal with the symptoms you are experiencing. Maybe you have been newly diagnosed with an autoimmune disorder and looking for ways to tame the inflammation that is ravaging your body. Whatever the reasons are, you have been given a reason to smile because you might finally have stumbled across a diet that may help manage and maintain your condition – the Autoimmune Protocol Diet (AIP diet).

What is the Autoimmune Protocol?

Whether you want to admit it or not, with the world in crisis due to a global pandemic, one thing is certain and that is that you have been forced to take a look at your overall health. For the better part of a year, we have been listening to the World Health Organization (WHO), doctors, epidemiologists, immunologists, and anyone with a medical degree talking about immune systems, viruses, and comorbidities. For those who do not have a medical degree and just regular, everyday folk, all the scientific explanations and information is overwhelming. Millions turned to the internet looking for ways to boost immune systems and stay virus-free.

The Autoimmune Protocol was created with the aim of improving the quality of life for all individuals. Whether you suffer from chronic disorders or not, the AIP is beneficial to everyone. The AIP focuses on retraining your mind, body, and soul by going back to basics. Diet or the food you eat is important to your body, but there is so much more happening behind the scenes that it is important to your overall health.

Lifestyle

There are two aspects to the Autoimmune Protocol; diet which involves food and nourishment, and lifestyle. You cannot do one without the other. The whole idea is to heal your body, and food alone cannot do that. Take stock of what is going on in your life. Look at some of the signs you simply dismissed as being part of everyday life. You will need to make some changes to your lifestyle, no matter how big or small. This does not only apply to the AIP diet, but to all people on whatever path they are on.

Stress

Stress affects everyone. Those that say they don't get stressed and they have no concerns, in my opinion, are in denial. Everyone worries about something whether it be about finances, work, or health. Yes, everyone worries about something, and being human, you tend to jump in and solve issues without thinking which creates even more tension. We are all human after all and it is in our nature to deal with issues alone. Do not be afraid to reach out and ask for help.

- Do not try to do everything alone, ask for help from family, friends, or coworkers.

- Do not be afraid to use that little two-letter word: NO. Make sure people understand your no answer.

- Surround yourself with positive people. Negative people can suck the energy out of you which increases your stress levels and you end up doubting yourself.

- Cut down on unnecessary stress at work. If you feel like you are drowning under all the work, take a lap around the office, do a couple of laps on the staircase, or head outdoors and get some fresh air.

Exercise

Exercise is important to any lifestyle. Some people have mobility issues due to their disorders or they are insecure about exercising in front of strangers. You do not need to go to the gym. Get the blood flowing by walking at a comfortable pace. Put on some music in the privacy of your home and away. Do yoga. Sweep a room in your house or vacuum. It is important to move and not give up because you think it will hurt. You set the pace. You are in control. This is your journey to healing.

Sleep

Your body needs sleep to function. Sleep deprivation plays a negative role in your health. You might be proud that you can go without sleep for two or three days. If you are not getting the right amount of sleep your body requires, you are putting your already compromised immune system at risk.

If you are a bad sleeper, try and change your bedtime habits. There are several options that you can put into practice to help you and probably some tips you have seen mentioned a few times. As a warning, some of these tips might not meet with your approval. Since this book is all about helping you manage your autoimmune disorders, you need to be open to making positive changes.

- Ditch the screens, all screens from smartphone to television, an hour before going to bed. No screens in bed. The temptation is real but fight it.

- Read a book before turning off the light.

- Put on some soothing music or a white noise machine.

- Essential oils in a diffuser.

- Go to bed at the same time every night.

- Set an alarm and stay in bed until your alarm goes off.

- Consistency is key in teaching yourself how to sleep again. Do not give up. Remember why you are doing this. Your health is important.

Fresh Air

Being outdoors, in nature, is beneficial to your health. Not only does it help with mental clarity and stress reduction, but it is also beneficial for your immune system. You will be soaking up the essential vitamin D which is excellent for your overall health. Ditch the screens and spend time outdoors. Go hiking, stroll around the neighborhood, or start a little garden in your backyard.

Diet

Our daily existence revolves around food and beverages. Whether you agree or not, you think about food more often than you think about how much money you have in your wallet. It is perfectly fine to think about food. It is completely normal to plan your evening meal at breakfast time. If you work a 10-hour day, you need to plan in advance. What you do not put as much thought into is what type of food or beverage you will be consuming. You know you are going to make burgers. There was not enough time to prepare the burgers from scratch, thank goodness for the box in the freezer. The burgers need some sweet potato fries but you did not have time to wash, peel, and cut them up – freezer to the rescue. What else do the burgers need? Oh yes, a creamy mushroom sauce, but there is absolutely no time to whip up a fresh batch. It is okay, there is a jar in the pantry. What about a bun for the burger? No, no buns. We are eating a healthy meal and as it is, you already have the fries, so you do not need bread as well.

We try to be conscious of what we put into our bodies. We listen to the conversations around the watercooler at work, or the body-conscious ladies working out at the gym. Without understanding their reasoning, you decide to implement your interpretation of what a diet should be. The intention is there but the execution is lacking because no one has explained how certain food affects your body, especially if you suffer from any number of autoimmune disorders. The Autoimmune Protocol was designed to look at the relationship food has with the immune system, your microbiome, regulating your hormones, and the healing of damaged tissues in your body.

Target Areas

Diet and lifestyle are important to our existence. What we consume plays a role in our lives, whether we are following a diet or doing our own thing. The same can be said for lifestyles, we can be taming it down by making sure we are in bed at 10 PM every night, or drinking and dancing at the club.

It is believed that there are four areas responsible for the autoimmune disorders, pain, and discomfort patients experience. The Autoimmune Protocol, diet, and lifestyle, will play an important part in each of the target areas to help you achieve your manageable lifestyle.

Nutrient Consumption

Your body needs nutrients to operate. Nutrients consist of vitamins, minerals, amino acids, and more. If you are not getting the correct nutrients or if you are nutrient deficient, you could be opening a door that would have a negative impact on your health. Typically, you would take supplements from the drugstore, or a more advanced way is by completing a survey and then being told what you would need. The best way to get all the nutrients in one sitting is by changing the way you look and think about food. When you change your diet and eat what is on your permitted food list, you will be cramming all the essential vitamins and nutrients into your immune system so that the healing can begin.

Digestive Happiness

Your body needs wholesome food that is free of corrosive additives that damage your intestinal lining. When your lining is damaged, it becomes compromised, inviting harmful bacteria to go exploring in channels where they should not be. Diet and lifestyle are important in maintaining a healthy balance between what you put into your body, and the activities you participate in to keep your immune system energized.

Hormone Balance

Your immune system and your hormone levels work together. Depending on the type of food you eat and the quantity, your hormones will be awoken and they will trigger the immune system into reacting. Diet and lifestyle are important factors in keeping the hormone levels regulated. Eat good food, sleep, fresh air, and less stress to keep your hormones from raging out of control.

Balancing the Immune System

The only way to regulate and restore a healthy balance in our immune systems is to change the way we think about food, what we put into our bodies, and how we cope with life. Yes, diet and lifestyle are important to our immune systems and contribute to our overall health and well-being. By following the AIP diet, you are allowing your immune system to heal itself.

Autoimmune Protocol Diet's Purpose

Throughout this journey, we have circled many different obstacles, made discoveries, and hinted at the relationship your immune system might have with food. You might know more about the immune system than you ever thought possible or you might be finding pieces of the puzzle that are just now being discovered. The AIP diet is a two-phase diet that will be explained in more detail in Chapter 8.

What you have learned thus far is that a healthy immune system produces antibodies that are intended to fight off harmful entities in your body. In an immune system that is over eager and produces more antibodies than is needed, those antibodies get confused and the good versus good battle follows. You also know that everything you consume has to go somewhere before it is expelled from your body. This is where what you eat and your lifestyle comes under the spotlight. It has been mentioned over and over, but every person's body is wired differently. No two people will have the same reaction.

Broken Walls

You do not tend to give too much thought into what modern-day convenience meal you are consuming, and this does not mean that you do not care. We are creatures of habit and the brain has been taught to see what we want it to see and everything around it is a blur. We forget, only to be reminded when our guts stage a protest, that everything that enters our body in the way of food, has to go somewhere. From the mouth to the anus, small and large intestines included, it is a long journey between the entrance and the exit. Along the way, there are various twists and turns.

Our digestive system is essential to our daily existence. The food gets broken down, analyzed, and processed like a production line in a factory. Sometimes the food we take in is not broken down properly and we can encounter a whole host of issues. The food that is not processed correctly will find cracks in the intestines and seep into the bloodstream. As discussed in the previous chapter, this is known as the leaky gut syndrome. The AIP diet wants to teach you how to retrain your body by starting over. In starting over, you need to cut out food that is harmful and abrasive to the digestive system.

By starting over, you are showing your digestive system that you are aware and that you acknowledge there is an issue and that you are going to be consciously making a change to patch up the cracks in the broken walls or lining. Remember, the AIP diet is not a cure for autoimmune disorders, but it can help you manage your symptoms.

No Quick Fixes

If you have to be honest with yourself, you were hoping this book would give you the answer you were looking for, and that is a quick fix for your autoimmune disorder. As much as I would love to tell you that yes, your autoimmune disorder can be cured, it would go against all my morals. Health is important to me. I do not want to give anyone false hope because I have seen firsthand, how debilitating autoimmune disorders can be. Never say never when it comes to hoping for a cure. You can hold onto the belief that someday, one of the millions of scientists will stumble upon a cure.

The Ups

Scientists have conducted several studies focusing on the relationship between the AIP diet and certain autoimmune disorders. The intention of these studies was to determine whether the AIP diet would improve the quality of life in patients when removing certain food types from their diet and changing their lifestyles. While most of the studies performed gave satisfactory conclusions, some tests were inconclusive and further testing would be required.

Researchers determined that changing the diet of patients with inflammatory bowel disease or the sub disorders, ulcerative colitis or Crohn's disease, would benefit and quality of life would be possible.

In a study performed on females between the ages of 20 to 45, who had been diagnosed with Hashimoto's concluded that following the AIP diet would improve their quality of life. There were no significant changes to the levels of the thyroid of the antibodies, but an indication that the inflammatory response in the body was decreased.

The Downs

As far as diets go, no matter which one you are following, there is a downside. This creates balance because, for some or other unknown reason, life cannot give you a break to enjoy good without experience bad.

The AIP diet was not created to make your life a misery. It was created to improve your quality of life by taming the inflammation that is attempting to take over your body. The AIP diet takes you through a rigorous cycle where you are retrained to change how your body accepts and processes food. This is the process of elimination. Everything that you love when it comes to food and beverages is removed from your diet.

You will be going back to the beginning and you are going to cleanse your body from the inside out by removing everything that is processed and has inflammation-inducing qualities such as potatoes, tomatoes, and refined sugar. This minute list is a very small crumb on the cookie sheet.

Due to the strenuous elimination cycle which lasts approximately 90 days, you become comfortable with this new way of eating that the thought of reintroducing food makes you break out in a cold sweat. You have to reintroduce food as your body will need to learn how to absorb and make use of the nutrients needed.

Two Diets, One Goal

You have been reading about the AIP diet, and you almost understand what this diet entails. To help you understand a little better, I am going to introduce you to the older brother, the paleo diet. It is believed that the paleo diet hails from the paleolithic age and that the name was originally the caveman diet. Whatever its origin or its name, it made its way to the 21st century. Many naysayers have classed the paleo as a fad diet. That means that it is a craze and as quickly as it has arrived, it will be disappearing again. I doubt that it will be going anywhere anytime soon because who doesn't want to follow a diet that scientists and researchers have picked and pulled apart to give you answers.

The paleo diet has been through the wringer since it arrived in our midst. There are those that say that you are doing more harm than good to your body by removing or restricting certain foods that are deemed to be vital for our health. In fact, scientists and researchers have weighed in ever so slightly, to say that by following the paleo diet, the benefits are great. If you are overweight and struggle with the typical overweight issues such as physical exhaustion or low energy, the paleo diet might be what you need. Other studies have whispered that following the Paleo way of life helps in managing the inflammation in certain autoimmune disorders such as psoriasis, inflammatory bowel disease, and multiple sclerosis.

The Paleo Way of Life

You spotted some trigger words that would make you believe that the paleo diet and the AIP diet are the same. They might have the same intentions by restricting what you eat, but they are slightly different. In a way, the paleo diet is a little more lenient and not as strict as the AIP diet.

The AIP diet eliminates dairy, eggs, legumes, grains, seeds, sugar, and everything that is processed such as oils, sauces, and lunch meats. For the full list of what is allowed and what is not, you can look at Chapter 7. The elimination list for the AIP diet looks very intimidating, but this is where one of the differences between the two diets pop up. The AIP diet has a reintroduction phase where you can slowly and calmly start adding food from your forbidden list and monitor your progress in the process. More to come in Chapter 8.

Paleo Food List

The paleo diet is slightly more forgiving in what you are allowed to consume. People who follow the paleo diet are more likely to follow it for the weight loss benefits. In addition to weight loss, there are the added benefits of reducing inflammation, heart disease, and blood sugar levels. The biggest differences between the two diets are what food is allowed to be consumed. Do not mistake the paleo list for the AIP list. The official AIP food guide is found in Chapter 7.

- Eggs

- Nuts

- Seeds

- Spices

- Tomatoes

- Potatoes

- Red wine

- Dark chocolate

- Tea

- Coffee

- Chilies

- Hot peppers

As you can see, the choices on the paleo diet offer a wider variety. People who follow the paleo diet do not have to count calories or macronutrients. It is believed that if following the approved lists and pulling the breaks when satiated, you will lose weight.

In Summary

Before we can move onto the part of the book you have been waiting for, we have to stop and ask ourselves a couple of important questions.

Are **YOU** ready to make changes that will positively affect **YOUR** health?

Are **YOU** ready to commit to changing **YOUR** ways for the better?

Are **YOU** ready to join forces with the Autoimmune Protocol diet and lifestyle?

You have to do what is right for you. You have a number of well-meaning friends and family who are eager to give advice, but their advice might not fit in with the AIP diet and lifestyle plan. It is your body and you have a choice. If you are feeling overwhelmed by all the information, find someone outside your immediate circle. There are social media groups and various online forums where you can get support for your specific disorder. You will know what you want to do. Make a commitment to yourself and hold yourself accountable for your actions. Remember, you are human and no one is perfect. If you are still feeling unsure, speak to your doctor.

Chapter 7:

AIP Diet Food Guide

Until now you have been reading about food that you should be avoiding, what you should be eating more of, and what you should be avoiding. You are probably wondering what you may or should be eating. All the information you have at your fingertips is pretty overwhelming. Reading about the various autoimmune disorders have you worried about your family members.

The AIP diet is not only for people with autoimmune disorders. You might have an uncle who has psoriasis and you have seen how this disorder caused him discomfort. He tried his best to hide these flaky skin cakes in blood, but you still saw it. The embarrassment he felt when people stared at him and pointed fingers, and then took wide steps to avoid getting close to him. The pain on his face was evident. There was no help or guidance for him in the 1980s when his skin started changing. No one told him what he should be doing or what he could do to manage the pain. Doctors gave him a water-based lotion and told him to use baby oil so that the skin would peel away without having to pick at the flakes.

Today you wish that you could call him up and tell him about the AIP diet. We have to appreciate modern-day science and the amount of work scientists are putting into their research. Some people are desperate and will try just about anything to manage the symptoms of their disorders. It was always an unspoken rule that food was not the enemy. You could choose to eat something but your choice had consequences.

Tomatoes are an excellent example of a choice with consequences. If you know you have ulcerative colitis, tomatoes are something that should be avoided like the plague. As delicious as a bright red, plump tomato looks, you know that you are setting yourself up for a couple of days of agony. You try to listen to that little voice in your gut that warns you to walk away. That tomato is taunting you. It is calling you by name. You try to be strong but the tomato wins. Is the pain from eating that tomato worth it? No, but it was really delicious. You made a choice and you have to suffer the consequences.

Why Food Guides Are Needed

Food guides or lists are designed to help you make good choices. Changes can be overwhelming for most people. The first thing people do when being introduced to a new diet or lifestyle is to look at what they should be consuming. Food guides are not meant to destroy your life; they are designed to help you make good choices to benefit your life.

There are hundreds of diets being circulated that claim to be the best. Some diets are created by some well-meaning sofa dieticians who have decided that they need to lose some weight. They experiment with different foods and, after a week of trying their diet, have dropped three pounds and are ready to share their tips with friends, family, or anyone that will listen. A diet cannot be created overnight. There is a process that goes into creating diets. This process can take months or even years before it is ready to be introduced to the market.

No one can force you to follow one specific diet. No one can force you into changing your ways with immediate effect. You need to be prepared and that is why food guides are important to any lifestyle change. You get to scrutinize the food lists of what you should be eating and look at what you should not be eating. Take the time to process the information you have been given. Mentally prepare yourself for a change. Create a shopping list with what you will need.

Remember that you have choices. You can choose to continue with your current lifestyle. Every choice comes with a consequence. Do not let your choices become consequences. Look at the tomato scenario again. Ask yourself if the pain, cramps, swollen joints, or reflux was worthwhile. The AIP diet is not meant to punish you. It is meant to help you to alleviate some of the symptoms you may experience. Eat clean. Eat food that will be beneficial to your health. As you will see when you reach the recipes at the end of this book, you can enjoy all your favorite foods by experimenting.

Think outside the box. Work through your elimination process. Do not give up, no matter how frustrated or defeated you may feel. There will be a very bright light at the end of the tunnel. Let us have a look at the food lists to see what is waiting for you.

Permitted Food List

The items mentioned in this list can be used freely. There are however some items listed in this list that have been mentioned in the 'occasional' list such as carrots, sweet potatoes, and fruit.

Vegetables

Most vegetables contain phytonutrients and fiber which are beneficial to our health.

- Artichokes

- Asparagus

- Avocado

- Arugula/Rocket

- Artichoke hearts

- Acorn squash

- All lettuce

- All mushrooms

- Brussel sprouts

- Butternut squash

- Beets

- Bok Choy

- Broccoli

- Carrots

- Cauliflower

- Celery

- Cassava

- Cabbage

- Cucumber

- Chicory

- Chinese cabbage

- Collard greens

- Dandelion

- Endive

- Fennel

- Jerusalem artichokes

- Kale

- Kohlrabi

- Leeks

- Mustard greens

- Onions

- Parsley

- Pumpkin

- Parsnips

- Radish

- Rutabaga

- Spaghetti squash

- Sweet potato

- Spinach

- Swiss chard

- Squash

- Turnips

- Turnip greens

- Taro

- Watercress

- Yellow squash

- Yam

- Zucchini

Fruits

Fruits contain fiber and antioxidants that safeguard our cells against possible damage. The recommended helpings are two to five servings a day. Fruit and vegetables contain fructose which is a form of natural sugar.

- Apples

- Apricots

- Blueberries

- Blackberries

- Bananas

- Cranberries

- Coconut

- Cantaloupe/sweet melon

- Cherries

- Dates

- Figs

- Citrus

- Grapes

- Guavas

- Honeydew melons

- Kiwi fruit

- Lychee

- Mangoes

- Nectarine

- Papaya

- Peaches

- Pears

- Passion fruit

- Pineapple

- Persimmon

- Pomegranates

- Plums

- Olives

- Raspberries

- Star fruit

- Strawberries

- Watermelon

Herbs

Herbs are the magic ingredient that adds an abundance of flavor to your meals. They contain phytonutrients which means that it helps protect your cells. Most herbs offer medicinal properties to help with inflammation, acts as a calming agent, or helps you sleep.

- Basil

- Bay leaves

- Chamomile

- Chives
- Cilantro
- Cinnamon
- Dill weed
- Cloves
- Lemon balm
- Garlic
- Ginger
- Lavender
- Horseradish
- Marjoram
- Peppermint
- Parsley
- Saffron
- Sage
- Rosemary
- Sea salt

- Spearmint

- Thyme

- Oregano

- Tarragon

- Turmeric

- Wasabi

- Lemongrass

- Lime leaves

Animal Protein

All animal protein is good to eat but preference is giving to grass-fed, wild-caught, and pasture-raised meat. Some diets put a 'forbidden' or "eat in moderation" label on animal protein. With the AIP diet, all animal protein is believed to have healing properties that are important to your overall health.

- Chicken

- Bison

- Turkey

- Lamb

- Pork

- Turkey

- Alligator

- Duck

- Venison

- Beef

- Wild boar

- Sheep/mutton

- Moose

- Pheasant

- Quail

- Elk

- Kangaroo

- Deer

- Snake

- Rabbit

- Veal

- Wild turkey

Offal/Organ Meats

Many might be gagging at the thought of eating organ meat of animals but these delicacies are the most nutritious of all the foods on these lists. They make the most delicious casseroles, stews, or pates. Experiment with them and savor each bite.

- Liver

- Kidney

- Bone marrow

- Brain

- Sweetbreads

- Rinds

- Skin

- Tongue

- Heart

- Tripe

- Blood

- Tail

Seafood and Shellfish

If nutritious is what you are after, look at your variety of fish. Preference should be given to wild-caught fish or fresh fish. Shell-fish and offal fall into the same nutritious category which is packed with nutrients.

- Fish

- Anchovies

- Cod

- Haddock

- Mackerel

- Mahi-mahi

- Red snapper

- Sardines

- Tuna

- Shark

- Trout

- Halibut

- Bass

- Eel

- Perch

- Salmon

- Haddock

- Rockfish

- Sole

- Turbot

- Grouper

- Shellfish

- Scallops

- Abalone

- Shrimp

- Clams

- Oysters

- Crab

- Mussels

- Lobster

Oils/Fats

Healthy fats are needed to keep you full so that you do not end up snacking or reaching for food that is not permitted. The fats also keep the inflammation levels in your body regulated, as well as provide smooth sailing for your nutrients to reach their destination.

- Palm oil

- Avocado oil

- Tallow/lard

- Chicken fat

- Olive oil

- Coconut oil

- Bacon fat

- Duck fat

Pantry Essentials

Every pantry needs the following items. When shopping for these products, make sure they do not contain additives that do not comply with the AIP diet guidelines.

- Apple cider vinegar

- Coconut flour

- Cassava flour

- Dried fruit

- Tapioca starch

- Tigernut flour

- Arrowroot starch

- Carob powder

- Tea

- Red wine vinegar

- White wine vinegar

- Balsamic vinegar

- Capers

- Gelatin

- Coconut water

- Coconut milk

- Coconut milk kefir

- Kombucha (sugar-free)

- Baking soda

- Coconut cream

- Plantain flour

- Water chestnut flour

- Green banana flour

- Cream of tartar

- Coconut aminos

- Gluten-free alcohol for cooking purposes

- Nutritional yeast

Fermented Products

Dairy-free fermented foods and live cultures are beneficial for your gut health. It is food for your microbiome and keeps healthy bacteria happy.

- Coconut kefir

- Water kefir

- Coconut yogurt

- Fermented sauerkraut

Forbidden Food List

This is the list that will tell you what you should avoid. For someone starting on the AIP diet, these foods are forbidden for a while. These items have been identified as being triggers for flare ups in the immune system. After ·following the AIP diet for a month, the reintroduction will start. There are various stages and guidelines that need to be followed. We will be looking at the elimination and reintroduction in the next chapter. Do not give up hope, as you might just be able to eat your cheese or oats at some point. Right now, all we need to focus on is getting you healthy and placing your disorder in quarantine.

When going through this list, you might be wondering why some of these items were mentioned as healthy alternatives when we were looking at the various autoimmune disorders. Those were the recommendations from dieticians and are not to be confused with the AIP diet.

Grains

- Rice

- Barley

- All varieties of wheat

- Corn

- Semolina

- Rye

- Durum

- Sorghum

- Wild rice

- Oats

- Millet

- Buckwheat

- Chia seeds

- Quinoa

Dairy

- Yogurt

- Cheese

- Cottage cheese

- Cream

- Butter

- Curds

- Whey

- Buttermilk

- Cream cheese

- Milk

- Dairy Kefir

- Sour cream

- Whipping cream

- Ice cream

- Frozen Yoghurt

Legumes

- Bean sprouts

- Black beans

- Edible bean pods

- Broad beans

- Calico beans

- Italian beans

- Black-eyed peas

- Butter beans

- Chickpeas

- Fava beans

- Cannellini beans

- Edamame

- Mung beans

- Lima beans

- Soybeans

- Tofu

- Split peas

- Lentils

- Kidney beans

- Pinto beans

- Peas

- Peanuts

- Tempeh

- Garbanzo beans

- Sugar snap peas

Vegetable Oils

- Sunflower oil

- Canola oil

- Grapeseed oil

- Palm kernel oil

- Peanut oil

- Rapeseed oil

- Soybean oil

- Palm olein

Ingredients Used in the Processing of Food

If you do not know what the meaning of the words on the labels is, then it is forbidden.

- Monosodium Glutamate (MSG)

- Xanthan gum

- Hydrogenated oil

- Artificial food colors

- Trans fats

- Textured vegetable protein

- Yeast extract

Sugars

This is a busy list with lots of different types of sugars and syrups. Certain sugars and syrups are allowed in moderation and will be mentioned in the next list.

- Treacle

- Rice bran syrup

- Refined sugar

- Stevia

- Sorghum syrup

- Agave and agave nectar

- Beet sugar

- Brown sugar

- Corn syrup

- Cane sugar

- Caramel

- Fructose

- Fruit juice

- Demerara sugar

- Barley malt

- Dextrin

- Glucose

- Muscovado sugar

- Raw sugar

- Monk fruit

- Golden syrup

Artificial Sweeteners

- Aspartame

- Stevia

- Xylitol

- Sucralose

- Saccharin

- Erythritol

Nuts and Oils

- Butters, oils, flours, and anything associated with nuts is not permitted.

- Almonds

- Walnuts

- Pecans

- Pine nuts

- Chestnuts

- Pistachios

- Peanuts

- Macadamia nuts

- Hazelnuts

- Brazil nuts

- Cashews

Seeds and Oils

As with the nuts list, anything made with seeds is not permitted.

- Chia

- Flax

- Coffee

- Hemp

- Pumpkin seeds

- Sunflower seeds

- Tahini

- Sesame

- Chocolate

- Cacao

- Poppy seeds

- Cocoa

Spices

- Fennel seeds

- Cumin

- Caraway

- Celery seeds

- Coriander

- Pepper

- Nutmeg

- Mustard

- Juniper

- Allspice

- Black caraway

- Fenugreek

- Cardamon

- Dill seed

Nightshades and Spices

- Potatoes

- Eggplant/brinjal

- Cape gooseberries

- Chili peppers

- Ground cherries

- Goji berries

- Hot peppers

- Sweet peppers

- Chili spice

- Tomatillos

- Tomatoes

- Tobacco

- Tamarillos

- Cayenne pepper

- Capsicum

- Garam masala spice

- Paleo ketchup

Eggs

- Chicken

- Duck

- Quail

- Goose

Alcohol

All alcoholic beverages are strictly forbidden.

- Beer

- Liquor

- Wine

- Whiskey

- Brandy

Miscellaneous

- Aloe vera

- Black pepper

- Elderberry

- Over the counter pain medication

- Psyllium husk

- Slippery elm

- Peppercorns

- White pepper

Occasional Food List

This list pales in comparison to the permitted and forbidden foods lists. While permitted, there is a limitation in place. For instance, the natural sweeteners are to be used for cooking purposes and not eaten with a spoon to satisfy some cravings.

Fructose

Fructose is a natural sugar found in fruit and some starchy vegetables, such as sweet potatoes.

Salt

Using too much salt is not beneficial to your health. Season your food with permitted herbs and salt-free spices. When shopping for your salt, choose coarse sea salt, Himalayan pink salt, or Celtic gray salt.

High Glycemic Fruit and Vegetables

There are various high glycemic fruit and vegetables that are naturally high in sugar and should be consumed a couple of times a week. These types of foods increase your blood sugar levels.

- Dried fruit

- Plantain

- Taro root

Fatty Acid Foods

Poultry and fatty meats are high in omega-6 polyunsaturated fats and should be limited to a couple of times a week.

Tea

Since you are being deprived of your coffee fix, you can enjoy three or four cups of tea a day. Black and green tea are permitted on the AIP diet.

Use in Moderation

- Coconut

- Honey

- Blackstrap molasses

- Maple syrup

- Saturated fat

In Summary

After reading through the lists, you might be wondering about the cost implications of purchasing all the food and condiments needed. The AIP diet does not require you to empty the bank. Start with the basics such as protein, vegetables, and fruit. At the end of the day, you are saving money by not buying convenience and junk food. As long as you have the basics in your pantry, you are good to go. If you feel that you are ready to put your big toe in the pond and experiment with your recipes, buy what you need and build up your new and improved pantry.

We will be looking at how the AIP diet works and the processes which are involved. If you are still sitting on the fence, hop on over to Chapter 8 to find out how this lifestyle change is going to work. I can almost guarantee that by the end of Chapter 8, you will be ready to start implementing changes and looking for the signup sheet.

Chapter 8:

Preparing for the AIP Diet

While researching the relationship between food and the immune system, I stumbled upon many diets. I am passionate about nutrition and the way people respond to different diets, lifestyles, and changes. I want to offer guidance and support. Naturally, when researching, you click on hundreds of links. These links have more links and each link leads somewhere. I found a support group on one of the social media platforms that were targeted at a specific lifestyle that includes a lot of this and not a lot of that. I am not going to throw this group under the bus because, from what I could see, it is quite a popular group. There also seem to be a lot more women in the group than men. By observing this group for a week, something struck me as being odd.

New members of the group were asking for an explanation or guidance on how they should prepare for the diet. No answer was given, but a link to the information was provided without further explanation. Either the admin of the group are lazy, or just tired of answering the same questions all day long. In my opinion, this is setting the person intending to follow the diet plan to fail. Meaning no disrespect to anyone, but I have come across men and women from all walks of life who need things explained simply without all the technical and scientific terms. If something was explained simply and in a language that could be understood, the more you will remember.

This chapter is going to explain all you need to know about the AIP diet, and what it involves. Unlike the social media group I hinted at, I will not be giving you a link and wishing you well as I move on. We started this journey together, and we will see it through right until the end. You will have me at your fingertips whenever you need to refresh your memory or need a little bit of encouragement when you are feeling low.

Stepping Stones

By now you are either excited to learn how your new way of life is going to work, or you are petrified at how you will react to the changes. You have seen the food lists, and the mere thought of not drinking coffee or eating a jacket potato with a (not so) healthy dollop of sour cream has you trembling. If you are going to follow the AIP diet to the letter, you will get to see your coffee or your sour cream potato again.

What you will be doing is healing yourself, that is the immune system, intestines, lines, joints, tissues, muscles, and organs. You will also be learning how to regulate your hormones and various other bodily functions, as well as managing pain and discomfort. What an amazing gift you are giving to your body. You decided to do this. No one, I hope, held a gun to food and threatened to blow it up if you did not change your ways. One of the secret rules to dieting or changing your lifestyle is that you need to do it for yourself. You are the most important person. If you are doing the AIP diet, or any other diet for your children, spouse, or partner, you are setting yourself up for failure. Do it with yourself in mind and if you have a bad day and eat something wrong, you hold yourself accountable, berate yourself and move on.

One, Two, Three — GO!

The AIP diet, as you know from all the sneak peeks, is a diet that works by way of a process of elimination. Three phases need to be followed to achieve the desired outcome.

- Elimination phase

- Reintroduction phase

- Maintenance phase

You do need to follow each of these phases in the order of how they appear. You cannot jump around between the phases and claim that the AIP diet did nothing for you. Each phase will be explained as we move through the sections.

I would not have embarked on this journey if I did not believe that there was hope for people like the young lady I mentioned in the introduction, or Marge. Watching people who struggle with mobility issues or skin conditions is heartbreaking. The look of embarrassment and defeat on their faces as they look around at the sea of faces looking at them is not a pretty sight. Let us get exploring!

The AIP Diet: Elimination Phase

There are two options for you to consider when starting the AIP diet. Instead of overwhelming yourself by just jumping straight in and going through shock at the sudden elimination of coffee, you can transition into the AIP diet by following the paleo diet. The reason for starting with the paleo diet is because it is not as restrictive and you will still be able to have certain food and spices before you cut them out. If you are confident that you have the willpower to power through any possible cravings, you may choose to go cold turkey.

Each of these transition processes has downsides which you should be made aware of. If you do plan to follow the paleo diet first, this could prolong your AIP journey. If you are opting to go cold turkey, you could be putting too much pressure on your immune system and it may cause you some negative responses due to the elimination of food you have eaten daily.

Purpose of Eliminating Food

This is a tough one to wrap your head around. You know what is good for you and know what you should be avoiding. This may seem cruel, especially cutting out coffee and chocolate, but there is a reason for the madness. The food on the forbidden list was tested by researchers who concluded that the items contained compounds that would be harmful to the digestive tract, as well as agitate the immune system by sending false sensors and alerting the antibodies of possible invaders in the body.

The food items went through a "vote of no confidence" as they were weighed up against their possible targets based on the damage they can cause to our bodies such as allergic reactions or inflammation properties. What you are aiming for when removing the processed food, seeds, nuts, legumes, grains, and so forth, from your diet, is to allow your body time to heal.

You might have people telling you that you are making the mistake by following such a restrictive diet and that you are being deprived of the vital nutrients to keep you healthy. Do not listen to these negative people. If you are doing the AIP diet correctly, you have spoken to your doctor or wellness nurse about your intentions. You are not being deprived of anything, when in fact, you are packing more nutrients into your body than you were before.

The Importance of Eating Nutrient-Rich Food

When you looked at your food guide lists, and as you have read through the lists a frown appeared when you spotted some of the items. The realization that you are being permitted to eat food that was taboo, makes you start to wonder what changed. The medical profession started taking notice of the value of the nutrients in the different food categories.

- Organ meats, all animals such as chicken, sheep, lamb, pork, and so forth.

- Vegetables, emphasis on colorful vegetables.

- Fish and shellfish.

- Fermented vegetables and fruit.

- Bone broth, full of collagen which is beneficial for skin, hair, and joints.

- Fats such as unprocessed oils and animal fats that you have cooked yourself.

These food groups are high in nutrients that are beneficial for healing or putting your immune system on the right track by giving it the fuel it needs.

Duration of the Elimination Phase

The duration of the elimination phase is not set in stone, but it is recommended that you stick to the plan anywhere from 30 to 90 days. If you feel that your symptoms are improving or have improved tremendously before the end of 90 days, you can start the reintroduction phase. It is important to remember that the elimination phase is not part of the long-term goal of the AIP diet. The whole concept behind the elimination phase is to give your body time to heal after removing all products that are deemed to be harmful or irritating to your microbiome, tissues, joints, or hormones.

The AIP Diet: Reintroduction Phase

When you are satisfied that you are not feeling any symptoms related to your autoimmune disorder, you can begin the process of reintroduction. Do not make the mistake of, when reintroducing food that you have not had for up to three months, going on some kind of binge-eating fest. You will need to take caution with what to eat, how much, and the protocol involved in reintroducing food.

It has been mentioned previously that by following the process of elimination, you are retraining your body. In a backhanded way, you can say that you are showing your body who is the boss by taking control. If, during the elimination phase you notice that some of your symptoms have lessened or have been put to sleep — remember, autoimmune disorders cannot be cured but you can go into remission and your symptoms could be decreased to a manageable level. If you reach this level and you feel that you have new symptoms, visit your doctor to get it sorted out. You might not need a lot of medication due to the effect of the AIP diet working its magic and easing your condition.

Reintroduction Process

You are going to need a food diary for the reintroduction phase. The reason behind this bit of advice is so that you can record your reaction to the food. If you keep track of what you are eating and how you react, you will have evidence to present to your doctor when you go for your physical.

During the reintroduction phase, please do not try to be the hero. If you have a negative reaction to any food you introduce, stop immediately, and continue with the elimination phase. If you are going to ignore the negative reactions, you are just undoing all the positive work you had done until that point. There is no rush to reintroduce food back into your system, but it has to be done eventually. As the keeper of your body, you will know when the time is right to start adding food again.

If you are feeling sick, stressed, lacking sleep or just generally out of sorts with everything, refrain from reintroducing food until you are feeling better or in a better space of mind. We have mentioned previously that diet and lifestyle work together. You cannot do one successfully without the other.

How to Reintroduce Food?

The recommendation process for reintroducing food is to introduce one piece of food every five to seven days. Remember to keep your diary close to monitor your reaction. If at any time you feel your symptoms coming on, stop the process and wait. This is not a race to see how quickly you can drink a glass of wine or have a cup of coffee.

There are different reintroduction phases that you can use but for our purpose, and not to make you seem like a hungry wolf. Here is a simple guideline you can follow when you start reintroducing your food.

1. Choose the one food item you have missed the most during the elimination phase. For the sake of using an example, let us assume you chose dark chocolate.

2. Break your chocolate into small pieces.

3. Place one small piece in your mouth and eat it.

4. Wait for approximately 15 to 2o minutes.

5. Take special note if you are feeling any pain, nausea, or any type of discomfort.

6. If symptoms are noted, stop eating.

7. If no symptoms are noted, take another bite of your chocolate.

8. Wait for approximately 15 to 20 minutes.

9. Again, record how you are feeling. If you are feeling any symptoms, stop eating immediately.

10. If no symptoms are noted, take a slightly bigger piece of chocolate.

11. Wait for approximately three hours.

12. During this long waiting period, take notes of how you are feeling.

13. If you are still not presenting any symptoms after three hours, incorporate the rest of your chocolate with your evening meal, like a chocolate sauce for your dessert or whatever you decide on.

14. That concludes the first day of the first item of the reintroduction phase.

15. Do not eat the potato again during the first week.

16. Do not pick another food during the five to seven days. Wait until the full time has passed before you introduce another food.

17. Continue to monitor your symptoms during the five to seven days.

If you show no symptoms on day seven, you have successfully reintroduced your first food item!

What Symptoms Should You Look Out For?

Watching your body like a hawk, waiting to see what symptoms you might develop can be very intimidating. You do not know what you should be feeling and if you do feel indifferent, you do not know if that is a symptom or your imagination.

Here are a few symptoms to look out for.

- Lack of energy

- Struggling to sleep

- Stomach cramps

- Painful joints

- Headaches

- Skin issues

- Nausea

- Coughing

- Sneezing

- Anxiety

You know your body and you are the best judge. If you display any of these symptoms or any that are not mentioned here, stop with the reintroduction and wait. Remember to keep notes of how you are feeling.

Reintroduction Food Stages

If you are overwhelmed and not sure which food to introduce first, consider taking it in stages. There are four different stages. Work through each stage until you have tried all the food in the group, remembering to keep notes of your reaction or any symptoms that might develop. If you have any allergies to any of the items in the stages, omit them. Do not, under any circumstances, put your health at risk. We have not come this far to have you end up with a nut or lactose allergy.

Stage One

- Egg yolks — no whites

- Seed fruit

- Oils made with nuts and seeds

- Grass-fed dairy ghee

- Coffee, in moderation

- Dark chocolate

- Peas such as snap and snow peas

- Beans

- Bean sprouts

Stage Two

- Seeds such as chia, sesame, and flax seeds

- All nuts

- Egg whites

- Coffee

- Butter

- Alcohol in moderation

Stage Three

- Eggplant/Brinjal

- Green/yellow sweet peppers

- Paprika

- Dried legumes such as lentils, split peas, and chickpeas

- Potatoes, peeled

Stage Four

- Chilies

- Jacket potatoes

- Tomatoes

- White rice

The AIP Diet: Maintenance Phase

Looking back at the whole process you went through to get to this point; you can smile with pride and pat yourself on the back. You accomplished what many said you could not. You might have had a couple of bumps along the way but you got through it. You had one clear vision and that was to take care of your damaged immune system. You are on the right road. It is important not to give up. You have come this far, and to give up will be heart-wrenching.

The maintenance phase is the last of the three phases. This phase is all about maintaining what you have done since the elimination phase and then the reintroduction. The reintroduction phase was rather insightful, as you could sift through the food items to see what triggered responses that agitated your autoimmune disorder. Whatever foods were eliminated can remain on the back burner until such time you are ready to try again. The maintenance phase is your personal diet. This is unique to you, based on what your body needs and requires.

You can make use of the AIP tools at any time you feel you are regressing and your symptoms are making a return. This is normal and to be expected. These things happen to keep us on our toes and make sure we are not too comfortable and in a groove that takes us back to our previous ways and habits. Make it a habit to keep your food diary updated. Note changes in your health. Identify symptoms, especially recurring symptoms. Visit your doctor for physicals and blood work to keep an eye on your disorder or condition.

Be an advocate for your body and health. Remember that lifestyle is part and parcel of your maintenance phase. Learn how to cope with stressful situations and walk away if you have to. Sleep, rest is vitally important to your overall health. Continue moving. Head off to the beach or the mountains, or just potter around in your garden. Speak to your plants, they will not judge you.

You can do anything you put your mind to. You have one life, make it count.

In Summary

This has probably been one of the most difficult experiences of your life, after being diagnosed with an autoimmune disorder. Retraining your body and listening to your body makes you realize that you can and will do better. Eliminating the food was not as hard as you thought and others tried to tell you. The hardest was adding food you liked to your diet again. It was daunting because you did not know what to expect, and yet you managed. The process does not stop there, it is an ongoing process. It is part of your daily life. Enjoy your new life!

You have been taught how to change your ways by making little changes. The biggest change might have been the part about getting sleep and getting rid of nighttime screens. I have to admit that putting the screens away, especially out of the bedroom, is quite a challenge but you adapt. If you do something and keep doing it, you are forming a new habit. Do not be afraid of changes. Embrace them. You have done a great job in making it this far. Get ready for the last couple of chapters which are going to take you on a culinary tour.

You are going to encounter food you thought you would never see again, sauces you would never be able to use, and treats you all but said goodbye to.

Chapter 9:

AIP Diet: Breakfast Ideas

Starting the day with a delicious, nutritious breakfast seems too good to be true. Considering your dietary restrictions, you are wondering whether you will be able to get through the day by drinking a glass of water. Lifestyle changes might seem daunting but they can also be fun. Experimenting with your food to make it palatable might seem like hard work but it shouldn't be. Feel free to experiment with the food you have at your disposal and put your own spin on the following recipes. All recipes were designed to be played around with.

All the recipes have been tailored with the elimination phase in mind. These recipes, across the following four chapters, can accommodate your reintroduction and maintenance phase.

Cereals

Breakfast Crunch

You want a crunchy breakfast cereal. You are missing your regular sugar-laden cereals. We heard you before you could ask. This recipe can be used for breakfast or as a snack. It can be stored in an airtight container and enjoyed without worrying about any repercussions to your disorder. At the end of the recipe, I will be including a list of optional extras. You can add and remove anything from the original recipe to suit your taste buds.

Time: 1 hour 20 minutes

Serving Size: 16 oz

Prep Time: 10 minutes

Cook Time: 1 hour 10 minutes

Ingredients:

- 2 ½ cups grated white sweet potatoes

- 2 cups coconut flakes, unsweetened

- 5 oz banana

- 2 ½ cups plantain, either chips or strips

- 1 tbsp cinnamon

- ¼ cup maple syrup

- Freshly ground sea salt to taste

Directions:

Part One

1. Preheat your oven to 325 F.

2. Add the grated sweet potatoes to a large mixing bowl.

3. Lightly crush the plantain chips or strips but be careful not to crush them to a powder.

4. Add the plantains chips to the sweet potatoes.

5. Grate your apple and using a kitchen towel, wring out the juice.

6. Add the apple to the mixing bowl.

7. Add the coconut flakes.

Part Two

1. Using your food processor, add the bananas and maple syrup.

2. Mix until you have a smooth consistency.

3. Add the cinnamon to the sweet potato, plantain, apple, and coconut mixture.

4. Add the banana and maple syrup to the mixture.

5. Mix well to ensure all the ingredients are evenly distributed.

6. Line your baking tray with parchment paper.

7. Turn the mixture out onto the baking tray.

8. Spread the mixture evenly over the tray and press it down.

9. Add freshly ground salt over the mixture.

Part Three

1. Put the baking sheet in the preheated oven and bake for 30 minutes.

2. After 30 minutes, remove the baking tray and turn the mixture over. It is okay if it breaks apart at this point.

3. Press the mixture down again and return it to the oven for 20 minutes.

4. After 20 minutes, remove the baking tray and turn the mixture over again.

5. Keep a watchful eye so that the edges do not burn.

6. Return the baking sheet to the oven and bake for 20 to 25 minutes.

7. During the period, stir the mixture approximately every 10 minutes.

8. Each time you stir, your mixing will agitate the mixture and break apart – this is what you want.

9. Remove your baking tray from the oven and allow the mixture to cool.

10. Once cool to the touch, it can be placed in an airtight container.

Optional extras:

This list will include dried fruit which should be chopped into smaller pieces or freeze-dried fruit.

- Banana chips

- Cherries

- Prunes

- Raspberries

- Raisins

- Strawberries

- Apricots

- Dates

- Figs

- Blueberries

- Fresh fruits

- Kiwi fruit

- Pomegranate seeds

- Kumquats

- Strawberries

Crunchy Flakes

Missing your favorite breakfast cereals? Here is an adaption you will want every day. It is so good that you can enjoy it as a snack. This recipe can be created in bulk and kept in an airtight container.

Time: 35 minutes

Serving Size: 5 servings

Prep Time: 15 minutes

Cook Time: 20 minutes

Ingredients:

- 2 cups banana chips, homemade or unsweetened store-bought

- 1 ½ cups coconut flakes

- ¼ cup coconut flour

- 2 tbsp gelatin granules

- ¼ cup honey

- ¼ cup of water

- ½ tsp salt

- 2 tbsp coconut oil

Directions:

1. Turn the oven to 350°F.

2. Line a baking sheet with parchment and grease with coconut oil.

3. Add banana chips and coconut flakes to the food processor and mix together until it resembles powder.

4. Add gelatin granules, coconut flour, and salt to the mixture and mix.

5. Add honey and water and mix until combined.

6. Turn the mixture out onto the baking sheet and press down.

7. Use a rolling pin or bottle to spread the mixture across the sheet.

8. Bake for approximately 10 minutes.

9. Remove from the oven and allow to cool for a couple of minutes.

10. Break or cut the baked mixture into small pieces that resemble bite-size flakes.

11. Return to the oven and bake for approximately 5 to 10 minutes.

12. Stir the pieces around the baking sheet to make sure they do not burn.

13. When a golden color has been reached, remove from the oven and allow to cool.

14. When cool, transfer to an airtight container for storage.

15. Serve with homemade coconut yogurt topped with fresh berries.

Vegetable Porridge

You might enjoy vegetables for dinner but you are not too sure about eating your vegetables for breakfast, especially not in the form of porridge. Do not knock it until you have tried it. People tend to get desperate when on a restrictive diet and crave all the food they are not supposed to consume for fear of a flare-up. You will mix a whole of everything together just to see what works and what doesn't. Food is very forgiving and there are no limits to your experimentations.

Time: 10 minutes

Serving Size: 2 servings

Prep Time: 10 minutes

Cook Time: 0

Ingredients:

- 1 large apple

- ½ a head of cauliflower

- Cinnamon to taste

- ½ cup of water or coconut milk

Directions:

1. Peel the apple, remove the core, and chop it into chunks.

2. Break the cauliflower into florets.

3. In a microwave-safe container or steamer, steam the cauliflower until soft.

4. Add the steamed cauliflower, apple chunks, cinnamon, and coconut milk or water into a blender.

5. Blend to a smooth consistency.

Carrot Porridge

Here we are again with another delicious vegetable breakfast porridge. You can make this in batches and pop them in the freezer. Breakfast on the go.

Time: 40 minutes

Serving Size: 4 servings

Prep Time: 10 minutes

Cook Time: 30 minutes

Ingredients:

- 1 small head of cauliflower

- 8 medium-sized carrots

- ½ tsp ginger powder

- ¼ tsp mace

- 1 tsp ground cinnamon

- 1 tsp vanilla powder

- 13.5 oz coconut milk

- 1 tbsp maple

Directions:

1. Wash and chop carrots into chunks.

2. Wash and floret cauliflower.

3. Add carrots and cauliflower to a large saucepan with water.

4. Steam for approximately 30 minutes or until soft.

5. Drain the water.

6. Add the carrots and cauliflower to the food processor.

7. Add coconut milk, maple syrup, cinnamon, mace, vanilla powder, and ginger and mix until smooth.

Optional extras:

- Berries

- Banana chips

- Fresh fruit

- A sprinkle of Breakfast Crunch or Crunchy Flakes

Breakfast Baked Goodness

Devilish Waffles

Waffles? Did someone say waffles? And you thought that your life as you knew it was over because of your new lifestyle. I warned you, where there is a will, there is a way. You do not ever have to feel that you are being deprived of your favorite foods. This meal is an ideal way to kickstart the day or even as a dessert.

Time: 15 minutes

Serving Size: 2 servings

Prep Time: 5 minutes

Cook Time: 10 minutes

Ingredients:

- 2 tsp gelatin granules

- 2 tbsp hot water

- 5 ½ tbsp coconut flour

- 1 cup cassava flour

- Pinch of salt

- ½ tsp baking soda

- ½ tsp cream of tartar

- 1 ½ tbsp solidified coconut oil

- 1/3 cup of hot water

- 2 tbsp honey

- Blueberries

Directions:

1. Sprinkle the gelatin granules over 2 tbsp of hot water and set aside.

2. Turn on the waffle maker to preheat.

3. Add the coconut flour, cassava flour, salt, baking soda, and cream of tartar into a mixing bowl and stir to evenly distribute the ingredients.

4. Melt the coconut oil.

5. Add the gelatin, honey, and coconut oil to the dry ingredients.

6. Add the hot water and stir to combine all the ingredients. The mixture will resemble a doughy consistency.

7. Measure out half of the dough onto the waffle maker and press down.

8. Cook until crispy.

9. Remove the waffle carefully before cooking the second one.

10. Drip with honey and serve with blueberries.

Perfectly Pancaked

Who does not like a pancake breakfast? The best is, this recipe is so versatile you can add spinach to the mixture for that extra goodness. These pancakes can be made in bulk, cooked, and into the freezer for those lazy mornings when cooking is the last thing anyone feels like doing.

Time: 20 minutes

Serving Size: 8 to 10 pancake rounds

Prep Time: 5 minutes

Cook Time: 15 minutes

Ingredients:

- ¼ cup of tapioca starch

- 1 cup cassava flour

- ¼ tsp sea salt

- ½ tsp baking soda

- 1 tsp cream of tartar

- 1⅛ cup of coconut milk

- ⅓ cup banana

- ½ tbsp apple cider vinegar

- 2 tbsp maple syrup

- 2 tbsp coconut oil

Directions:

1. Add the tapioca starch, cassava flour, sea salt, baking soda, and cream of tartar to a mixing bowl, and combine.

2. Mash the banana.

3. Add coconut milk, mashed banana, apple cider vinegar, and maple syrup to the blender and blend till smooth.

4. Add the dry ingredients to the mixture and blend to a smooth consistency.

5. Heat a skillet on medium.

6. Add coconut oil and spread to cover the skillet.

7. Using a ladle, spoon one or two spoons of the mixture onto the skillet, size depending on how big you want your pancakes. Repeat until the skillet is full.

8. Cook for approximately three minutes, or until bubbles appear.

9. Flip the pancakes and cook for a further three minutes.

10. Serve and enjoy with Saucy Chocolate Delight, dairy-free yogurt, or fresh fruit.

Not the Regular Hash Browns

Hash browns are typically prepared with potatoes which are not good for those with autoimmune disorders or anyone that has a carbohydrate intolerance. You might be craving hash browns, especially with your homemade sausage, you no longer have to dream. While we are substituting the potatoes for sweet potatoes, you can still enjoy your hash browns without feeling guilty or worrying about a flare-up of your disease. These hash browns can be enjoyed alone or as part of a side dish.

Time: 20 minutes

Serving Size: 2 servings

Prep Time: 10 minutes

Cook Time: 10 minutes

Ingredients:

- 1 large or 2 small sweet potatoes

- Salt to taste

- 2 tbsp ground arrowroot

- 2 tbsp coconut oil

Directions:

1. Peel the sweet potatoes.

2. Grate or shred the sweet potatoes.

3. Turn the sweet potatoes onto a kitchen cloth and wring out excess water.

4. Add the sweet potatoes to a mixing bowl and add the salt and arrowroot.

5. Melt the coconut oil on a large skillet.

6. Add the sweet potatoes to the skillet and spread evenly to cover the surface.

7. Cook for approximately 10 minutes, depending on the thickness until it is soft and lightly browned. Be careful not to burn.

8. Alternatively, if you want to make miniature hash browns, heap spoons full onto the skillet and cook until brown. Caution not to burn.

A Taste of Greece

You do not have to hop on a plane to fly to Greece to enjoy a delicious pita or flatbread in the comfort of your home. Bread you might be wondering. Bread is strictly a no-no because of the gluten and carbohydrate content. Do not worry, the experiments are not over just yet. In addition to showing you how to make your very own guilt-free pita bread, I will include an accompaniment that you can enjoy on the side.

Time: 25 minutes

Serving Size: 5 servings

Prep Time: 10 minutes

Cook Time: 15 minutes

Ingredients:

- 1 cup of cassava flour

- 1 ¼ cups coconut flour

- 1 tbsp garlic powder

- 1 tsp mixed herbs, dry or fresh

- 2 tsp baking soda

- 2 tsp cream of tartar

- Salt to taste

- 1 tbsp nutritional yeast

- 3 tbsp gelatin granules

- ½ cup piping hot water

- 3 tbsp lukewarm water

- 3 tbsp hot water

- 2 tbsp olive oil

- Fresh ground salt

Directions:

1. Turn on the oven to 350 F to preheat.

2. Add nutritional yeast to piping hot water and stir to dissolve.

3. Sprinkle gelatin granules over lukewarm water.

4. Add the hot water and stir until completely dissolved.

5. Add the gelatin and olive oil to the nutritional yeast mixture and stir the mixture well.

6. Add the cassava flour, coconut flour, garlic powder, baking soda, cream of tartar, salt, and herbs to a mixing bowl.

7. Stir to combine the dry ingredients.

8. Add the gelatin, olive oil, and yeast mixture to the dry ingredients and mix together with a spoon.

9. The mixture should resemble dough. If too dry, add 4 tbsp boiling water and continue mixing until a dough ball is formed.

10. Section the dough into five equal balls.

11. Flatten the balls between your hands.

12. On a lined baking tray, lay the flattened dough and shape it to resemble an oval shape.

13. Place the baking tray in the preheated oven and bake for 12 to 15 minutes.

14. Halfway through the bake, rotate the tray.

15. Remove from the oven and allow to cool.

16. Sprinkle some ground salt.

Lemon Berry Bliss

You have noticed a trend while going through the recipes and you might have come to the conclusion that being on a restrictive diet may not be that bad after all. Here we have a delicious lemon fruity muffin to start the day off right. Make in bulk, pop in the freezer, and grab one or two as you run out the door to go to work or sitting in the carpool lane. One teaspoon of vanilla extract may be added to the mixture when you reach your reintroduction or maintenance phase. There are enough flavors without the vanilla but everyone has a personal preference.

Time: 35 minutes

Serving Size: 10 muffins

Prep Time: 15 minutes

Cook Time: 20 minutes

Ingredients:

- ½ cup of coconut milk

- ¼ cup freshly squeezed lemon juice

- 5 tbsp honey

- 3 tbsp coconut oil

- 1 tbsp lemon zest

- ¼ cup of arrowroot flour

- ⅔ cup of coconut flour

- ⅛ tsp sea salt

- 1 tsp baking soda

- ¼ cup of water

- 1 tbsp gelatin granules

- ¾ cup blueberries

Directions:

1. Turn the oven to 350°F.

2. Prepare your muffin trays with parchment paper or cupcake liners.

3. Melt the coconut oil.

4. Add coconut milk, lemon juice, coconut oil, honey, and lemon zest to a mixing bowl.

5. Using a whisk or handheld mixed, combine until a smooth consistency.

6. Add arrowroot flour, coconut flour, salt, and baking soda to a clean mixing bowl.

7. Stir to combine the dry ingredients.

8. Using a large spoon, add the dry ingredients to the wet ingredients.

9. Mix well before adding more of the dry ingredients.

10. Continue the process until the dry ingredients have been added.

11. Set aside.

12. Add the water to a saucepan and turn it on low.

13. Carefully sprinkle the gelatin over the water and leave for a couple of minutes.

14. Increase the heat to medium and allow the gelatin to melt.

15. When melted, whisk the gelatin mixture until aerated.

16. Add the gelatin water to the prepared batter.

17. Whisk rapidly to combine.

18. Add the blueberries and carefully mix.

19. Fill the parchment or cupcake liners with the batter until ¾ full.

20. Place the muffin tray in the oven and bake for approximately 20 to 25 minutes.

21. Use a toothpick to see if the muffins have cooked through, the toothpick comes out clean.

22. If not cooked through, continue baking in increments of 5 minutes until ready.

23. Remove from the oven and allow to cool.

Meaty Breakfast

Homemade Sausage

If your idea of breakfast was going to one of the fast-food restaurants on the way to work for a couple of sausage breakfasts, this recipe will be an excellent addition to your AIP diet journey. This recipe calls for beef but can be substituted for any ground meat you prefer such as turkey, chicken, or pork. Making this recipe in bulk will cut down on preparation time. Simply make your mixture, portion your patties, and pop them into the freezer. Whenever you feel like a sausage breakfast, remove it from the freezer the night before and place it in the refrigerator to thaw overnight. There are no more excuses for not starting the day with a delicious homemade breakfast.

Time: 30 minutes

Serving Size: 4 large patties depending on the size you make

Prep Time: 10 minutes

Cook Time: 20 minutes

Ingredients:

- 1 lb ground beef but can be substituted for the meat of choice

- 2 tsp fresh sage finely sliced or 2 tsp ground sage

- ½ tsp ground mace

- ½ tsp garlic powder

- Salt to taste

- 1 to 2 tbsp of permitted fats such as animal fat or coconut oil

Directions:

1. Add the sage, garlic powder, mace, and salt to the ground beef and mix together to ensure the spices are evenly distributed.

2. Take a handful of the sausage mixture and form it into a hamburger patty.

3. Using a skillet, add your oil and turn the stovetop to medium-high.

4. Place the patties on the skillet with caution.

5. Cook on each side for between 8 to 10 minutes.

6. As an alternative to frying, you could bake it in the oven for between 15 to 20 minutes at 400°F.

7. Serve with leftover salad or vegetables.

Dinner for Breakfast Casserole

This delicious meal can be enjoyed at any meal. It is something you can prepare in advance and portion out for a quick meal when you are pressed for time or for those days when you do not feel like making breakfast.

Time: 45 minutes

Serving Size: 1 large serving

Prep Time: 10 minutes

Cook Time: 35 minutes

Ingredients:

- 4 tbsp avocado oil
- 2 chicken breasts
- 4 cups of chopped spinach
- ½ a cauliflower
- 2 thinly sliced carrots

- 1 medium-sized thinly sliced onion

- 2 tbsp freshly chopped parsley

- 2 tbsp freshly squeezed lemon juice

- 1 cup of coconut cream

- Salt to taste

Directions:

1. Turn the oven to 400°F.

2. Prepare a large casserole dish with 1 tbsp of avocado oil.

3. Using a large frying pan, add the rest of the avocado oil.

4. Add the chicken and onions to the frying pan and brown.

5. In a large mixing bowl, add the spinach, chopped cauliflower, carrots, coconut cream, parsley, and lemon juice.

6. Add the chicken and onions.

7. Add salt and combine well.

8. Add the mixture to the prepared casserole dish.

9. Place in the preheated oven and bake for 35 minutes or until the chicken is cooked through and the vegetables are al dente.

Savory Breakfast Muffins

Not really feeling the sweet and fruity breakfast, not to worry, we have you covered. This savory muffin will fit the requirement for tasty, delicious, nutritious and it will definitely check all the boxes. The recipe calls for sweet potato puree which you can find in the Breakfast Extras section of this chapter. Make in bulk and freeze for the days when you have an early morning appointment or no inspiration to cook.

Time: 40 minutes

Serving Size: 9 muffins

Prep Time: 15 minutes

Cook Time: 25 minutes

Ingredients:
- ¼ cup extra virgin olive oil
- ½ cup of applesauce, sugar-free
- ½ cup plus 3 tbsp sweet potato puree
- ¼ cup of tiger nut flour

- ¼ cup of tapioca starch

- ¾ cup of cassava

- ½ tsp of sea salt

- 1 tsp of onion powder

- 1 tsp of garlic powder

- 1 tsp baking soda

- 1 tbsp apple cider vinegar

- 2 tbsp hot water

- 1 tbsp gelatin granules

- 8 0z raw bacon

- ¼ cup chives

Directions:

1. Turn the oven to 350°F.

2. Line muffin trays with parchment paper or liners.

3. Wash and chop chives.

4. Heat a frying pan over medium heat and add bacon.

5. Cook until crispy.

6. Remove from heat and allow to cool.

7. Add applesauce, sweet potato puree, and olive oil to a mixing bowl.

8. Mix to combine.

9. Add the tapioca starch, cassava flour, tiger nut flour, baking soda, onion powder, garlic powder, and sea salt.

10. Stir to distribute evenly.

11. Add the wet ingredients to the dry ingredients.

12. Mix well to make a smooth batter.

13. Add gelatin granules, apple cider vinegar, and hot water to a bowl.

14. Whisk the mixture together until gelatin has dissolved and you have a foamy mixture.

15. Chop up the crispy bacon.

16. Add bacon and chives to the batter.

17. Fold the gelatin mixture into the batter, taking care not to overmix the batter.

18. Fill the liners with batter.

19. Place in the oven to bake for 25 minutes or until cooked through.

Faux Egg and Bacon

What is breakfast without bacon and eggs? Oh, wait, eggs are taboo during the elimination phase of the AIP diet. Do not despair, here is a recipe that will tease the taste buds into believing it is having eggs.

Time: 40 minutes

Serving Size: 2 servings

Prep Time: 10 minutes

Cook Time: 30 minutes

Ingredients:

- 1 small head of cauliflower

- 6 thick slices of bacon

- 1 tsp of coconut aminos

- 2 tbsp water

- ⅛ tsp turmeric powder

Directions:

1. Turn the oven to 400°F.

2. Using a baking sheet, line with parchment paper.

3. Cut the head of cauliflower into large rounds or steaks.

4. Place bacon and cauliflower rounds on the baking sheet.

5. Add water, coconut aminos, and turmeric to a bowl and whisk until combined.

6. Using a basting brush, baste the cauliflower with the mixture.

7. Place the baking sheet in the preheated oven and bake for approximately 20 minutes.

8. Remove from the oven when cooked.

Breakfast Extras

Dairy-Free Yogurt

This yogurt can be used for your Breakfast Crunch, as a meal on its own, or as a base for your side dishes.

Time: 5 minutes

Serving Size: 4 servings

Prep Time: 5 minutes

Cook Time: There is no cooking time but the resting time is between 24 to 48 hours

Ingredients:

- 1 15 oz can of coconut milk

- 2 probiotic capsules

Directions:

1. Separate the cream from the water once the can is opened.

2. Place the milk and cream into a glass container.

3. Mix the cream and milk to break up lumps.

4. Add the powder from the probiotic capsules.

5. Using a clean ceramic spoon, combine the probiotic powder with the milk mixture. Do not use a metal spoon.

6. Depending on how thick you prefer your yogurt, you may use the leftover coconut water.

7. Cover the container with a cheesecloth or kitchen towel and secure it with an elastic band.

8. Leave it on the counter, away from direct sunlight.

9. Allow it to stand for between 24 to 48 hours.

10. Test the yogurt mixture until it tastes like yogurt.

11. Once you are satisfied that your mixture tastes like yogurt, place the lid on and store it in the refrigerator.

12. Storing in the refrigerator will ensure the yogurt thickens.

Dairy-Free Tzatziki

We are heading off to Greece again. I could not leave you with a Greek-style bread and not give you something to scoop on top of it. This accompanying treat can be used as a side dish or as a dip at a dinner party. Whatever you decide on doing with it, enjoy this delicious guilt-free dip with your breakfast, lunch, dinner, or snack.

Time: 15 minutes

Serving Size: 2 cups

Prep Time: 15 minutes

Cook Time: No cooking time

Ingredients:

- 1 ½ cups of coconut yogurt

- 1 medium cucumber

- 1 ½ tbsp freshly squeezed lemon juice

- 1 tbsp finely chopped dill

- 2 cloves of finely chopped garlic

- ½ tsp sea salt

Directions:

1. Wash the cucumber.

2. Top and tails the cucumber and slice it in half lengthwise.

3. Remove the seeds.

4. Grate the cucumber.

5. Put the cucumber on a kitchen towel and wring out the water until a clump of cucumber remains.

6. Add the dried cucumber to a bowl.

7. Add the yogurt, lemon juice, garlic, dill, and salt to the cucumber.

8. Combine the mixture well.

9. Depending on how thick or watery you like your tzatziki, you can add some of the cucumber water to the consistency you prefer.

10. Chill in the refrigerator until you are ready to use it.

11. For presentation purposes, you can sprinkle some chopped dill and/or olive oil.

This 'n That Red Smoothie

You might not be the breakfast-eating type of person but you do like to start your day with something to tide you over to the next meal. This might be the perfect recipe for you. It is full of delicious goodness and if you squint your eyes, this smoothie might resemble a red velvet cake mixture.

Time: 10 minutes

Serving Size: 1 large serving

Prep Time: 10 minutes

Cook Time: No cooking time

Ingredients:

- 1 medium-sized banana

- 1 large beet that has been cooked

- ½ cup full fat coconut milk

- 1 tbsp carob powder

- ½ cup crushed ice

Directions:

1. Remove the skin of the beet and chop it into small pieces.

2. Add the pieces of beet, banana, carob powder, coconut milk, and crushed ice to a blender.

3. Blend the mixture until there are no more bits.

4. As an optional extra, you can add some whisked coconut cream.

Saucy Chocolate Delight

Craving chocolate but not ready to indulge in the real deal? Here is a guilt-and dairy-free recipe that was designed with you in mind. Drizzle over your pancakes, waffles, or fruit salad to enjoy. Chocolate sauce can be stored in the refrigerator for up to five days.

Time: 10 minutes

Serving Size: 4 servings

Prep Time: 5 minutes

Cook Time: 5 minutes

Ingredients:

- ½ cup of coconut milk

- 2 tbsp maple syrup

- 1 tbsp arrowroot

- 2 tbsp carob powder

- Pinch of sea salt

Directions:

1. Add coconut milk, maple syrup, arrowroot, carob powder, and sea salt to a saucepan.

2. Whisk together to combine.

3. Warm the mixture over medium heat.

4. Continue whisking until thickened.

Sweet Potato Puree

This creamy puree can be used as a side dish or for part of recipes. The original recipe calls for an Instant Pot to be used, but not everyone has one, so we will be going old school by boiling the sweet potatoes on the stovetop like Grandma used to.

Time: 25 minutes

Serving Size: 6 serving

Prep Time: 5 minutes

Cook Time: 20 minutes

Ingredients:

- 2 lb sweet potatoes

- 1 ½ cup beef, pork, or chicken bone broth, or alternatively vegetable stock

- ½ tsp sea salt

Directions:

1. Wash, peel, and cube the sweet potatoes.

2. Add broth or stock to a saucepan and add cubed sweet potatoes.

3. Cook for approximately 15 to 20 minutes until soft.

4. Pour the mixture into the blender and add the sea salt.

5. Blend until smooth.

Chapter 10:

AIP Diet: Lunch Ideas

Eating a wholesome, nutritious meal at lunchtime will help you get through the midday slump. The days of ordering sandwiches laden with saturated fats, processed meat, and high in carbohydrates are over. You have already seen what your breakfast options could look like, now imagine what would be on offer for lunch. By eating a nutritious meal, your blood sugar levels will be stabilized, give you energy, and keep you focused. The recipes are not limited to set meal times and can be switched around to be enjoyed at any meal.

Salads

Crunchy Green Goodness

When you think about diets, you are transported back in time to when it was believed that eating copious amounts of lettuce, tomatoes, and cucumber were healthy. Those were the salads that became our worst enemies. It is time to change your mindset and envision nothing but delicious crunchy goodness.

Time: 10 minutes

Serving Size: 1 large serving

Prep Time: 10 minutes

Cook Time: No cooking time

Ingredients:

- 1 romaine lettuce

- 1 Granny Smith apple

- 10 grapes

- 1 stem of celery

- 2 tbsp coconut cream

- 1 tsp freshly squeezed juice

- Fresh ground salt

Directions:

1. Wash and chop the lettuce.

2. Thinly slice the apple.

3. Thinly slice the celery at an angle.

4. Cut the grapes in half.

5. Mix the coconut cream and fresh lemon juice to make the dressing.

6. Add salt to the dressing and well.

7. Add the lettuce, apple, celery, and grapes to a bowl.

8. Add the dressing to the salad and mix well to coat.

Something Fishy Salad

Adding a protein takes your salad to the next level. If salmon is not for you, you can replace it with pan-fried or grilled chicken breasts.

Time: 5 minutes

Serving Size: 2 servings

Prep Time: 5 minutes

Cook Time: No cooking time

Ingredients:

- 8 oz thinly sliced smoked salmon

- 4 to 5 oz mixed salad greens

- ½ cup blueberries

- 2 tbsp olive oil

- 1 tbsp balsamic vinegar

Directions:

1. Rinse the salad greens and pat dry.

2. Chop the salad greens.

3. Rinse the blueberries.

4. Add the salad greens and blueberries to a bowl.

5. Mix the olive oil and balsamic oil together.

6. Drizzle the dressing over the salad and mix around until coated.

7. Dress two plates with salad.

8. Place smoked salmon on top of the salad.

Bacon Brussels Sprouts Salad

Love it or hate it, Brussels sprouts have caused quite some fights or differences of opinions in many households. Children are traumatized by these little globes because it was used as a bargaining tool for getting dessert or staying up an extra hour. The most common way to eat Brussels sprouts was by boiling them in water and served with butter, salt, and pepper. Thankfully, times have changed and experiments with food came along.

This recipe combines flavor, tartness, sweetness, crispness, and crunch to kick the taste buds and make us want more. This salad can be enjoyed as a standalone meal or as a side dish with your dinner.

Time: 20 minutes

Serving Size: 4 servings

Prep Time: 10 minutes

Cook Time: 10 minutes

Ingredients:
- 1 ½ lb Brussels sprouts

- 8 oz bacon

- ¼ tsp cinnamon

- ¼ tsp sea salt

- ⅓ cup olive oil

- ⅓ cup coconut flakes

- ¾ dried apricots

- 2 tbsp freshly squeezed lemon juice

Directions:

1. Wash the Brussels sprouts.

2. Depending on your preference, you can leave your Brussels sprouts whole, chopped, or shredded/shaved.

3. Finely dice the bacon.

4. Place diced bacon in a hot pan.

5. Cook for approximately 10 minutes or until crispy.

6. Drain the bacon and set aside to cool.

7. Chop the apricots.

8. In a small mixing bowl, add olive oil, fresh lemon juice, cinnamon, and salt.

9. Whisk the dressing until combined.

10. Drizzle the dressing over the Brussels sprouts.

11. Mix well to ensure the dressing is coating the Brussels sprouts.

12. Add apricots, coconut flakes, and bacon pieces.

Protein Madness

Simply Delicious Burger

Happy days are here. Here, you have a succulent burger which is prepared with a whole lot of goodness and promises to keep you coming back for more. This burger is versatile and can be served with any toppings of your choice. One bite of this burger and you will forget that you ever frequented your local fast-food restaurant. If you do not like beef, you can substitute it with ground pork, chicken, or turkey. Meal preparation can be made easier if you prepare the burger mixture in bulk, portion them out, and pop them in the freezer for the days you do not feel like cooking. Your burger meal can be accompanied by cauliflower rice and the Crunchy Green Goodness salad, or sweet potato friends made with the correct oils.

Time: 30 minutes

Serving Size: 2 servings

Prep Time: 15 minutes

Cook Time: 15 minutes

Ingredients:

Rice

- ½ a cauliflower

- 1 tbsp coconut oil

- Season to taste

Burger

- ½ lb ground beef

- 1 tbsp garlic powder

- 1 tbsp onion powder

- Ground sea salt to taste

Gravy

- 1 onion thinly sliced

- +/- 15 white button mushrooms

- 2 garlic cloves thinly sliced

- 2 tbsp arrowroot powder

- 1 cup of beef broth

- 2 tbsp coconut oil

Topping

- 1 small beet

- ½ an avocado

- 2 tbsp chopped parsley

Directions:

Rice

1. Cut up the cauliflower and place it in the food processor.

2. Mix until the cauliflower resembles rice.

3. Melt the coconut oil in a frying pan over moderate heat.

4. Add the cauliflower to the pan and cook until soft for approximately 8 to 12 minutes.

5. Remove from the heat, season with salt, and set it aside.

Burger

1. Put the ground beef in a mixing bowl.

2. Add the garlic powder, onion powder, and salt to the ground beef.

3. Mix well to combine the spices.

4. Divide the ground beef mixture into two balls and flatten to form your burger.

5. Heat the coconut oil in a frying pan.

6. Place the patties on the frying pan and cook to your preference.

7. When cooked, remove from the heat and remove the patties from the pan.

8. Set aside to keep warm.

Gravy

1. Using the same pan, add extra coconut oil if needed.

2. Add the thinly sliced onions and sauté until soft.

3. Add the garlic.

4. Chop the mushrooms and add to the pan.

5. Cook the onions, garlic, and mushrooms until caramelized.

6. Add ¾ of beef broth to the mixture and allow to simmer.

7. Use the remaining broth to mix the arrowroot powder.

8. Add the arrowroot mixture once the mixture in the pan has reduced.

9. Cook for a further 1 to 2 minutes until you have a thick gravy.

Topping

1. Peel and slice the avocado.

2. Remove the skin from the beet and cut into small cubes.

3. Dressing your plate

4. Spoon a generous helping of cauliflower rice onto your plate.

5. Place your burger on the bed of cauliflower rice.

6. Ladle gravy over your burger.

7. Top with avocado slices and beet cubes.

8. Sprinkle parsley.

Optional Extra Toppings

- Pineapple rounds

- Green olives

- Mandarin oranges

- Carrots

Guilt-Free Chicken Bites

If you are craving chicken nuggets, look no further. Change is hard for everyone, especially when you feel as if you cannot ever eat your favorite 'junk' food. There are ways to replicate any meal. With an addition of this and an exclusion of that, I can almost guarantee that your meal will be tastier than the original and the biggest bonus is that it is completely guilt-free.

Time: 40 minutes

Serving Size: 4 servings

Prep Time: 15 minutes

Cook Time: 25 minutes

Ingredients:

- ½ cup coconut flour

- 2 tsp of permitted dried herbs

- 1 lb filleted chicken breasts

- ½ tsp salt

- ¼ cup avocado oil

- Pour avocado oil into a spray bottle

Directions:

1. Preheat the oven to 400°F.

2. Add the coconut flour, salt, and herbs to a bowl and mix well.

3. Slice the chicken into squares or strips.

4. Add the chicken to the avocado oil and mix until the chicken is coated.

5. Roll the chicken pieces in the coconut flour, herbs, and salt until covered.

6. Place the chicken pieces on a baking tray.

7. Spray with avocado oil.

8. Bake for approximately 12 minutes.

9. Turn the chicken pieces over and spray with avocado oil.

10. Continue baking for approximately 12 minutes.

Sweet Potato Surprise

If we cannot have normal potatoes, we improvise and opt for the next best root vegetable which is the sweet potato. Sweet potatoes can make any meal stand out. It is naturally sweet and healthy. The two best combinations without compromising your health. This recipe is a twist on the original baked potato and stuffed with all the goodness our bodies need. The surprise pops out when you combine the various flavors. Sink your teeth into this delicious flavor-packed meal.

Time: 1 hour and 10 minutes

Serving Size: 4 servings

Prep Time: 1 hour

Cook Time: 10 minutes

Ingredients:

- 4 medium-sized sweet potatoes

- 3 tbsp lard

- 5 oz brown mushrooms

- 2 or 3 cloves of garlic

- 1 medium-sized red onion

- 1 tbsp freshly chopped oregano

- ½ cup chopped green olives

- ½ bunch of chopped kale

- 6 anchovy fillets

- 2 cans of sardines

- Freshly chopped parsley

Directions:

1. Turn the oven on to 400°F.

2. Wash the sweet potatoes.

3. Prick sweet potatoes with a fork.

4. Place on a baking sheet and bake for approximately 1 hour.

5. Melt the lard in a large pan.

6. Thinly slice the onion and add to the pan.

7. Cover the pan and allow the onion to sweat over low heat for approximately 6 to 8 minutes.

8. When the onions are soft and see-through, stir the mixture and continue cooking for approximately 3 to 4 minutes until they turn a golden color.

9. Mince the garlic.

10. Rinse the anchovy fillets.

11. Add the garlic, oregano, and anchovy fillets to the onions.

12. Add the kale and olives to the mixture and cook for 3 to 4 minutes. Kale will wilt.

13. Add the sardines and break into bite-sized chunks while warming.

14. Add the parsley.

15. Stir everything together.

16. Remove the baked sweet potatoes from the oven.

17. To serve, slice the sweet potatoes lengthwise, add ½ tsp of lard, and spoon the mixture on top of the sweet potato.

A Taste of Asia

If you cannot have traditional Asian cuisine, we have to improvise. Add a splash of this and a dash of that, close your eyes, and put your tastebuds to the test. That is what we will be doing now. For the purpose of this recipe, instead of soy sauce, we have to use coconut aminos, fermented coconut palm sap. If you are unable to find this product, you can add onion powder and maple syrup. If you want it a little saltier, add sea salt until you are satisfied with the end result.

We know that Asia is well known for serving meals with noodles but due to, you know, certain dietary restrictions, we will be improvising a little more. Beef can be replaced with pork or chicken breasts.

Time: 30 minutes

Serving Size: 2 servings

Prep Time: 10 minutes

Cook Time: 20 minutes

Ingredients:

- 10 oz beef

- ½ onion

- 10 garlic cloves

- 1 large piece of ginger

- 2 tbsp cilantro

- 1 large zucchini

- 2 tbsp avocado or coconut oil

- 2 tbsp coconut aminos or substitute

Directions:

1. Thinly slice the onion.

2. Slice or cube the beef.

3. Finely chop the garlic.

4. Dice the ginger.

5. Chop the cilantro.

6. Shred the zucchini.

7. Heat the avocado or coconut oil in a large pan.

8. Add and sauté the onions.

9. Add the beef.

10. Add the coconut aminos or substitute.

11. Cook until the beef is tender. At this point, you can cover your pan to speed the process along.

12. Add the garlic and ginger and cook for approximately 5 minutes.

13. In a separate pan, bring water to boil and add the zucchini.

14. Boil for 2 to 3 minutes and drain.

15. Add the zucchini noodles to a bowl and top with the beef mixture.

16. Sprinkle cilantro.

Soul-Warming Chili Without the Burn

On a cold winter's day, while the snow is falling to the ground, all you want is something that will warm your insides. We know that the real chilies are part of the nightshade family, so we cannot use them but the next best thing is to imagine that you are eating a traditional chili con carne. This meal will, without a doubt, tick all the boxes and more to warm your stomach and soul, and keep you coming back for seconds. If you do not like beef, you can substitute it with any meat of your choice.

Time: 60 minutes

Serving Size: 4 servings

Prep Time: 15 minutes

Cook Time: 1 hour and 15 minutes

Ingredients:

- 1 lb ground beef

- 3 cloves garlic finely chopped

- 1 medium-sized red onion

- 2 tbsp olive oil

- 1 carrot

- 2 beets

- Approximately 20 white button mushrooms

- 1 tsp ground turmeric

- Salt to taste

- 2 cups beef broth/stock

- 2 small sweet potatoes

- Fresh parsley

Directions:

1. Peel and boil/roast the sweet potatoes.

2. When soft, mash the sweet potatoes and set aside.

3. Add the olive oil to a pan and heat.

4. Peel and chop the red onion.

5. Add the onion to the pan and sauté until soft.

6. Peel and dice the carrots and beets.

7. Chop the mushrooms.

8. Add the chopped garlic, carrots, beets, and mushrooms to the onion.

9. Fry the vegetables until almost caramelized.

10. Add the ground beef and turmeric.

11. When the beef has browned, add beef stock/broth and allow it to boil.

12. Reduce the temperature and bring to a simmer on low.

13. Partially cover the pan with a lid and cook for 45 to 50 minutes.

14. If there is too much liquid, remove the lid and increase the heat until the liquid reduces.

15. Add salt to taste.

16. Dressing your plate

17. Spoon the mashed sweet potato onto your plate.

18. Ladle a hearty helping of mock chili over your mashed sweet potatoes.

19. Sprinkle with parsley.

Noodle Soup

This recipe is a spin on ramen noodles without the noodles. This is a nutritious meal that will keep you fueled up until your next meal. Experiment with the permitted flavors. Change the protein to suit your preference. You are the chef and this recipe is your guideline.

Time: 15 minutes

Serving Size: 4 servings

Prep Time: 5 minutes

Cook Time: 10 minutes

Ingredients:

- 1 tsp coconut oil or lard

- 5 oz smoked bacon or pancetta

- 3 chicken breasts

- ½ tsp ground ginger

- 15 brown mushrooms

- 3 carrots

- 2 large zucchinis

- 2 cups spinach

- 3 spring onion stems

- 3 cups chicken stock/broth

- Salt to taste

- Bunch of cilantro

Directions:

1. Place a large saucepan on the stovetop and heat on medium.

2. Slice the bacon/pancetta and add to the saucepan.

3. Slice the mushrooms.

4. Wash, peel, and slice the carrots.

5. When the bacon/pancetta has browned, add sliced mushrooms and carrots to the pan.

6. Add ground ginger.

7. Stir to combine.

8. Slice the chicken breasts into thin pieces.

9. Add chicken to the saucepan.

10. Add the chicken stock/broth.

11. Add sea salt.

12. Simmer on low for approximately 5 minutes.

13. Cut the zucchini into thin strips that resemble noodles.

14. When the chicken is cooked through, add the zucchini strips to the saucepan for approximately 2 minutes.

15. Thinly slice the spring onion stems and add to the saucepan.

16. Stir the mixture.

17. When serving, place generous helpings of the chicken, zucchini, and vegetables into soup bowls.

18. Ladle the remaining broth over your chicken, zucchini, and vegetables.

19. Wash, dry, and roughly chop the cilantro and sprinkle over your soup.

Lunchtime Soups

Wholesome Butternut Soup

Not everyone wants to crunch or chew their food every day, so what better way to get in some nutrient-rich that requires heating and sipping. This recipe has everything that is needed to warm the stomach and soul on a cold winter's day. Make in bulk and portion out for a quick and easy meal.

Time: 1 hour and 10 minutes

Serving Size: 4 servings

Prep Time: 30 minutes

Cook Time: 40 minutes

Ingredients:

- 2 large onions

- 2 garlic cloves

- 1 large butternut squash

- 4 tbsp extra virgin oil

- 3 cups of homemade bone broth

- ½ cup of coconut milk

- 1 tbsp fresh tarragon

- 1 tsp sea salt

- 2 tbsp fresh lemon juice

Directions:

1. Preheat the oven to 350°F.

2. Peel the butternut and chop into cubes.

3. Coat the butternut with 2 tbsp extra virgin olive oil.

4. Add ½ tsp of salt and mix to distribute evenly.

5. Line the roasting pan or baking sheet with parchment paper.

6. Place butternut on the roasting pan or baking sheet and roast for approximately 25 minutes, until soft.

7. Peel and chop the onion.

8. Peel and mince the garlic.

9. Wash and chop the tarragon.

10. Add olive oil to a large saucepan and heat.

11. Add onions and garlic to the olive oil and sauté until cooked, not browned or burned.

12. Add roasted butternut to the saucepan.

13. Pour in bone broth and coconut milk.

14. Allow to heat without boiling.

15. Add salt and tarragon.

16. Add the soup mixture to the blender in batches and blend together until smooth.

17. Repeat until the contents of the saucepan have been blended.

18. Pour the contents from the blender back into the saucepan.

19. Heat over low heat.

20. Add the lemon juice and stir well.

Easy Bone Broth

Bone broth can be made by using any bones. It can be eaten as it or added to recipes to enhance flavors, as well as boost your nutrients. Overall, bone broth has excellent healing powers for the body as it contains collagen that is helpful for skin elasticity, helps the joints, and heals damaged tissues. It is a long process, but well worth the wait.

Time: 12 hours and 15 minutes

Serving Size: 12 servings

Prep Time: 15 minutes

Cook Time: 12 hours

Ingredients:

- Any bones

- Leftover juices, stray permitted vegetables — just about anything from a previously made roast or meaty meal

- 1 large onion

- 1 or 2 celery stalks

- 1 large carrot

- ½ tsp sea salt

- 1 bay leaf

- Depending on the size of your crockpot, enough water to reach within one inch from the top.

Directions:

1. Peel and chop the onion.

2. Chop the celery.

3. Peel and chop the carrot.

4. Add bones and leftover juices and vegetables to the crockpot.

5. Add the onions, carrots, celery, sea salt, and bay leaf to the crockpot.

6. Fill the crockpot with water.

7. Cook on low heat for up to 12 hours.

8. After 12 hours, remove all the bones and chunks of vegetables.

9. Using a sieve, strain the broth to ensure there are no stray bits of bones, vegetables, and leaves.

10. When cooled, dispense the broth to containers and store it in the refrigerator.

Hearty Vegetable Goodness

This hearty soul-warming soup was adapted to be AIP friendly. It contains a whole lot of goodness without the guilt and worries about how your immune system will react. In fact, the readaptation encompasses everything you are looking for as it is jam packed with nutritious vegetables and nutrients necessary to allow your immune system to have its own party. If making a large batch, portion out and freeze.

Time: 1 hour and 15 minutes

Serving Size: 6 servings

Prep Time: 15 minutes

Cook Time: 1 hour

Ingredients:

- 1 tbsp lard

- 6 oz sweet potato

- 12 oz carrots

- 6 oz parsnips

- 8 oz onions

- 3 garlic cloves

- 1½ cups of bone broth or vegetable stock

- Sea salt

- 1 small bunch of parsley

- 5 bay leaves

- 4 or 5 sprigs of fresh thyme

- 1 cup of coconut milk

Directions:

1. Peel and chop sweet potato, carrots, parsnips, and onion.

2. Peel and chop garlic.

3. Wash and chop parsley.

4. Wash the thyme.

5. Add the lard to a large saucepan and melt over medium heat.

6. Add the chopped carrots, onions, parsnips, sweet potato, and garlic and steam for five minutes.

7. Add the bone broth to the vegetables.

8. Add the bay leaves, thyme, and salt.

9. Bring the mixture to a boil.

10. When boiling, cover the saucepan and reduce to low, and simmer for approximately 20 minutes or until vegetables are soft.

11. Remove the thyme and bay leaves.

12. Transfer the vegetables to a blender and purée.

13. Add coconut milk and continue blending until you have a smooth consistency.

14. Ladle out generous helpings into bowls and garnish with chopped parsley.

Lunch Bakes

Guilt-Free Lasagna

If you are craving a pasta bake but have no idea how to indulge your craving, look no further. Here we have a gluten- and dairy-free mock pasta recipe that will satisfy the cravings. There is life after gluten products, and all it takes is a little bit of creativity and imagination to make it all come together. This is another one of those meals that can be prepared in bulk and frozen in portions.

Time: 1 hour and 25 minutes

Serving Size: 9 servings

Prep Time: 1 hour

Cook Time: 25 minutes

Ingredients:

- 4 large zucchinis

- 1 medium-sized onion

- 3 medium-sized carrots

- 2 garlic cloves

- 12 oz white button mushrooms

- 1 lb ground beef, pork, chicken, or turkey

- 2 beets

- 2 tbsp coconut aminos

- 2 tbsp red wine vinegar

- Fresh ground sea salt

- 2 tbsp olive oil

Directions:

1. Slice the zucchini, lengthwise, into ¼ inch thick slices.

2. Liberally sprinkle sea salt and lay on cooling racks.

3. Allow to sweat for 1 hour.

4. Turn the slices over every 20 minutes.

5. Dry the strips with a paper towel after an hour and set aside.

6. Preheat the oven to 350°F.

7. Peel and dice the carrots, onions, beets, and garlic.

8. Slice the mushrooms.

9. Using a large pan, heat the olive oil.

10. Add the diced onions and garlic and fry until soft but not browned.

11. Add the carrots, mushrooms, beets, and ground meat to the onions and garlic.

12. Cook until the meat has browned and the liquid has been reduced.

13. Add the red wine vinegar and coconut aminos.

14. Stir to combine all the flavors.

15. Add salt to taste.

16. Using a baking dish, assemble the lasagna by placing a layer of zucchini, topped with meat.

17. Repeat until all the meat and zucchini have been layered.

18. Cover the baking dish with aluminum foil and bake for 20 minutes.

19. Remove the aluminum foil and return to the over for a further 5 to 10 minutes.

Juicy Gluten-Free Chicken Pie

When you imagine a chicken pie, you envision the crispy pastry that encases the delicious filling. Until now, you never imagined eating a pie because, in your soul, you know that your stomach will be arranging a protest and invite all it's friends to protest along with it. Never fear, this will be a calm protest that will be enjoying every mouthful of pie you put in your mouth. Your intestines will be doing some dance moves as the food moves along slowly to its destination. What is not to love? It is crammed full of vegetables and a whole lot of creamy goodness. This pie can be enjoyed with a serving of lettuce and/or cauliflower rice.

Time: 1 hour and 5 minutes

Serving Size: 6 servings

Prep Time: 20 minutes

Cook Time: 45 minutes

Ingredients:

Pie filling

- 1 lb chicken breasts

- 2 tbsp coconut oil

- 1 tsp sea salt

- 1 medium onion

- 2 garlic cloves

- 1 cup of broccoli cut in florets

- 1 cup of diced carrots

- ½ cup of chopped celery

- 1½ cups of chicken bone broth

- ½ cup of coconut milk

- 1 tsp dried sage

- 2 tsp dried thyme

- 2 tsp arrowroot powder

Crust

- 3 to 4 tbsp coconut flour

- 1¼ cup and 2 tbsp cassava flour

- 1 tbsp gelatin granules

- ⅓ and ¼ cup of coconut oil

- ¼ cup and 2 tbsp water

- ¼ tsp sea salt

Directions:

Pie filling

1. Using a deep pie dish, grease with coconut oil.

2. Heat coconut in a large saucepan over medium heat.

3. Cube the chicken breasts.

4. Add the chicken cubes and salt to the saucepan.

5. Saute until cooked.

6. Remove from the saucepan.

7. Peel and dice the onion.

8. Peel and mince the garlic cloves.

9. In the same saucepan, add the onions and saute for 4 to 5 minutes, until soft.

10. Add garlic, celery, broccoli, and carrots.

11. Saute until the vegetables are tender, not too soft.

12. Add arrowroot powder and mix to incorporate evenly.

13. Add the chicken bone broth, coconut milk, sage, and thyme.

14. Mix well to combine all the flavors evenly.

15. Reduce the heat to slow and allow to simmer until the sauce has thickened.

16. Return the chicken to the mixture and stir well.

17. Add the mixture to the pie dish.

Crust

1. Turn the oven to 400°F to preheat.

2. Add coconut flour, salt, gelatin granules, and cassava flour to a missing bowl.

3. Add the coconut oil in solid form and combine the dry ingredients.

4. Add water and mix until the mixture resembles a doughy consistency.

5. Lightly flour the surface of the worktop with cassava flour, and turn the dough onto the worktop.

6. Lightly flour your rolling pin and roll the dough into a large circle.

7. The circle should be about ¼ an inch bigger than the pie dish.

8. Using flour to coat your hands, pick up the pie dough and carefully place it over the chicken filling, covering the pie dish.

9. If your crust has tears, you can pinch them together to seal the crust.

10. Pinch the sides together to cover the pie dish.

11. Score the crust to allow the steam to escape when baking.

12. Place the pie dish in the preheated oven and bake for approximately 20 to 25 minutes or until the edges of the crust are turning golden brown.

13. Remove the pie dish from the oven and allow to cool before serving.

Lunch Extras

Hey Pesto

Pesto can be used to complement most meals. Craving pasta but options are limited? Make your zucchini noodles by simply slicing them into thin strips and cooking in boiling water for 5 minutes. Drain and add your pesto, and you are good to go. This pesto recipe can be stored in an airtight container in the refrigerator for four days.

Time: 15 minutes

Serving Size: 4 servings

Prep Time: 10 minutes

Cook Time: 5 minutes

Ingredients:

- ¼ cup olive oil

- 1 cup fresh basil

- ½ cup flat-leaf parsley

- 3 garlic cloves

- 1 tbsp freshly squeezed lemon juice

- 2 tsp yeast flakes

- Salt to taste

Directions:

1. Add 1 tsp olive oil to a pan.

2. Peel and chop the garlic.

3. Add to the pan and fry until slightly golden.

4. Remove from the heat.

5. Wash and dry basil leaves.

6. Wash and dry parsley.

7. Using a food processor, add basil leaves, parsley, yeast flakes, and olive oil.

8. Add warm garlic.

9. Blend the ingredients to a smooth consistency.

10. Add salt and lemon juice.

11. Blend again to mix everything.

12. Store in an airtight container.

Magic Ketchup

As tomatoes are not favorable for our disorders, we have to improvise yet again. All you want is a hamburger and fries with ketchup. It is doable.

Time: 60 minutes

Serving Size: 12 servings

Prep Time: 10 minutes

Cook Time: 1 hour and 5 minutes

Ingredients:

- 1 large carrot

- 2 medium beets

- 2 tsp olive oil

- 2 tsp honey

- ½ tbsp red wine vinegar

- 1 cup of water

- Sea salt to taste

Directions:

1. Wash and peel the carrot and beets.

2. Dice the carrot and beets.

3. Over medium heat, add the olive oil, carrots, and beets.

4. Cook until caramelized and soft.

5. Pour in water and allow to boil.

6. Lower the heat, cover the pan, and simmer for approximately 1 hour.

7. Remove from the heat when the carrots and beets are soft.

8. Add red wine vinegar and honey.

9. Stir well.

10. Add sea salt to taste.

11. Set the mixture aside to cool.

12. When cool, add the mixture to a food processor and blend until smooth.

13. Transfer the mixture to an airtight container and keep in the refrigerator for up to four days.

Chapter 11:

AIP Diet: Dinner Ideas

Dinnertime is that time of the day, after a long day at work, running errands, or taking the children to various after school activities, that you do not want to think about creating a meal. Dinner is the last full meal of the day, the one that will tide you over until you start the next day over with breakfast. Until now, breakfast and lunch have featured some ideas that could easily be used at any meal. An added bonus is that all the meals are suitable for any time of the day.

Most of the meals thus far are versatile and open for experimentation. There are no limits. As a subtle reminder at this point, all these recipes are based on the ingredients allowed during the elimination phase of the AIP diet. While some of the original recipes had ingredients that were not AIP friendly, I adapted them to include suitable substitutes. As you start the reintroduction phase and are successful, you will be adding more variety in the form of spices, items from the nightshade family, and much more. Remember to make enough so that you can build up a stock supply for those days when you do not feel like cooking.

Let us have a look at what your dinner fairy has found for you. Bon appetit.

Palate Teasers

Fried Coconut Shrimp

A quick and easy, and let us not forget, crunchy goodness to start off the dinner chapter. These delightful crunchy shrimp can be enjoyed as a starter and enjoyed as is, or you can dunk them in your Dairy-Free Tzatziki, Magic Ketchup, or No-Fuss Mayo.

Time: 10 minutes

Serving Size: 2 servings

Prep Time: 5 minutes

Cook Time: 5 minutes

Ingredients:
- ½ cup of coconut flakes
- 2 tbsp coconut flour
- Approximately 1 cup of coconut oil
- 7 oz shrimp

- Sea salt to season

- 1 lime

Directions:

1. Put the coconut oil in a deep saucepan and heat.

2. Put coconut flour and coconut flakes in a mixing bowl and combine.

3. Put the shrimp in the coconut flour and flakes and coat well.

4. Carefully place the coated shrimp in the hot oil.

5. Fry for approximately two minutes.

6. Remove from the oil with a slotted spoon and place on kitchen towels to drain.

7. Slice the lime into wedges.

8. Serve the shrimp while warm, with lime wedges on the side.

Bacon Packages

Bacon is a favorite for any meal. These Bacon Packages are easy to make and are a combination of smoky, sweet and crispy. They are ideal as a starter before your main course, or as an addition to a dinner party platter.

Time: 40 minutes

Serving Size: 2 servings

Prep Time: 10 minutes

Cook Time: 30 minutes

Ingredients:

- 8 bacon rashers

- 2 medium-sized pears

Directions:

1. Turn the oven to 400°F.

2. Wash the pear.

3. Cut into quarters and remove the seeds.

4. Line a baking sheet with aluminum oil.

5. Wrap each quartered pear with the bacon rashers.

6. Place the wrapped bacon on the baking sheet.

7. Bake in the preheated oven for approximately 30 minutes, or until crispy.

8. Remove from the oven.

Beet Carpaccio

For a light, refreshing appetizer, Beet Carpaccio seemed like the ideal palate cleanser before diving into a main meal. Carpaccio can be made with beef, but for the sake of this recipe, vegetarians do not have to think about what they can use as substitutes.

Time: 10 minutes

Serving Size: 2 servings

Prep Time: 10 minutes

Cook Time: No cooking time

Ingredients:
- 7 oz beets
- 1½ tbsp extra virgin oil
- 1 tbsp apple cider vinegar
- 1 tbsp fresh chopped parsley
- Salt to taste

Directions:

- Rinse the beets.

- Peel the beets.

- Thinly slice the beets using a knife or a mandolin slicer.

- Arrange the sliced beets on a serving platter.

- Drizzle apple cider vinegar and olive oil over the slices of beets.

- Season with salt.

- Garnish with chopped parsley.

- Can be eaten once prepared, or can be left overnight for the apple cider vinegar to tenderize the beets.

Main Course

Creamy Smothered Meatballs

Meatballs are a firm favorite in many households. Typically, meatballs are swimming in tomato sauce and served on a bed of spaghetti. Unfortunately, due to circumstances out of your control, you cannot eat pasta and tomato sauce. But, in true AIP fashion, the recipes have been adapted to accommodate you. This recipe could possibly beat the traditional meatballs out of the ballpark with its creamy, nutritious goodness.

Time: 1 hour and 10 minutes

Serving Size: 4 servings

Prep Time: 30 minutes

Cook Time: 40 minutes

Ingredients:

Meatballs

- 1½ lb ground lamb, beef, turkey, chicken, or pork

- 1 small onion

- 2 or 3 garlic cloves

- 2 tbsp pumpkin puree

- 2 tsp avocado oil or olive oil

- ¼ cup of fresh chopped dill

- Sea salt

Mushroom sauce

- 3 tbsp avocado oil or olive oil

- 1 large shallot

- 2 garlic cloves

- 10 oz white button mushrooms

- 1 cup of coconut milk

- 1 cup of chicken bone broth

- Sea salt

- ¼ cup of fresh chopped dill

Cauliflower Mash

- 1 large cauliflower

- 4 to 6 tbsp rendered bacon fat

- Sea salt

Directions:

Meatballs

1. Peel and dice the onion.

2. Peel and mince the garlic.

3. Heat the oil in a frying pan and add onions.

4. Cook onions for approximately six minutes over low heat, until soft, not browned.

5. Stir in the minced garlic, and cook for approximately one minute.

6. Remove the onion and garlic from the pan and allow to cool.

7. Transfer the ground meat of choice to a large bowl.

8. Add the cooled onion and garlic mixture to the ground meat.

9. Add the pumpkin puree and chopped dill.

10. Using a large wooden spoon or your hands, combine everything together.

11. Make 16 to 18 small- to medium-sized balls.

12. Using the frying pan you used for the onions and garlic, add avocado or olive oil.

13. Place the meatballs into the frying pan.

14. Do not overpopulate the frying pan, a second batch might be needed.

15. Fry the meatballs on medium for approximately 15 minutes.

16. Turn them to ensure an even coloring of brown, not crispy or burnt.

17. Remove from the heat and set aside.

Mushroom sauce

1. Slice the shallot and mushrooms.

2. Mince the garlic cloves.

3. Add oil to a saucepan and heat.

4. Add the shallot and cook for approximately five minutes on low until see-through. Do not brown or burn.

5. Add the sliced mushrooms and minced garlic.

6. Cook on medium-low heat.

7. Stir to avoid the shallot and/or garlic burning.

8. Increase the heat to medium and add chicken broth and still to incorporate the juices.

9. Add the coconut milk and simmer for approximately seven to eight minutes.

10. The liquid should reduce by a third.

11. Pour the contents of the saucepan to a blender.

12. Blend until smooth.

Cauliflower mash

1. Wash and cut the cauliflower into chunks.

2. Add water to a saucepan and bring to boil.

3. Add the cauliflower chunks and cover with the lid.

4. Allow to steam for approximately eight minutes.

5. Remove from the saucepan and drain.

6. Add the steamed cauliflower to the food processor.

7. Add the rendered bacon fat and salt.

8. Blend until smooth.

9. Add more salt if necessary.

Serving Suggestion

1. Place the meatballs in a serving dish and cover with the mushroom sauce.

2. Garnish with chopped dill.

3. Dress the plate with a generous helping of cauliflower mash.

4. Top with meatballs and mushroom sauce.

Creamy Chicken Curry

As we are well aware, some of the really good spices that make the aromatic curries are in the no-go zone for the time being. By now, these restrictions have been easy to exclude due to the adaptation of the recipes to suit your dietary needs. This Creamy Chicken Curry is no exception. It is full of flavor and aromas that will have you believing you are eating the real deal but without that tangy bite. You can enjoy your Creamy Chicken Curry with cauliflower mash, cauliflower rice, or zucchini noodles as found in recipes throughout the previous three chapters.

Time: 1 hour and 25 minutes

Serving Size: 12 servings

Prep Time: 25 minutes

Cook Time: 60 minutes

Ingredients:

- 26 oz of chicken breasts
- 4 large parsnips
- 2 large sweet potatoes
- 1 large onion
- 2 stalks of celery
- 2 large cloves of garlic
- 3 cups of broccoli
- 3 tbsp liquid coconut oil
- 1 tsp garlic powder
- 1 tsp onion powder
- 1 tsp ground ginger
- 3 tbsp sea salt
- 1 tsp turmeric powder
- 1 tsp ground cinnamon
- 2 cans of coconut milk
- 1 cup of chicken bone broth

- 2 stalks of lemongrass

- Fresh coriander

Directions:

1. Turn the oven on to 350°F.

2. Wash, peel, and cube the sweet potatoes and parsnips.

3. Wash and chop the broccoli.

4. Peel and finely slice the onion.

5. Wash and finely dice the celery stalks.

6. Peel and mince the cloves of garlic.

7. Cut the chicken into cubes.

8. Add the sweet potatoes and parsnips to a mixing bowl.

9. Add 1 tbsp coconut oil, garlic powder, onion powder, 1 tbsp sea salt, turmeric powder, ground ginger, and ground cinnamon to the sweet potatoes and parsnips.

10. Stir well to evenly distribute the spices.

11. Turn the contents of the mixing bowl out into an oven dish and place in the preheated oven.

12. Cook for approximately 25 minutes.

13. The mixture will not be fully cooked but it does allow the flavors to activate.

14. Add 1 tbsp of coconut oil to a large saucepan and heat over medium heat.

15. Add onions and celery and cook until see through.

16. Add the minced garlic and cook for about two minutes.

17. Add the chicken cubes to the onion, celery, and garlic mixture.

18. Cook for seven minutes.

19. Add the broccoli and remaining sea salt.

20. Stir to combine everything.

21. Peel the lemongrass, remove the ends, and knock with a heavy object, meat tenderizer, or back of a knife to unleash the flavor.

22. Pour the coconut milk, chicken bone broth, the roasted sweet potatoes and parsnips, and lemongrass stalks to the saucepan.

23. Allow the mixture to boil.

24. Reduce the heat to simmer.

25. Cover the saucepan, and cook for approximately 15 minutes.

26. Remove the lid of the saucepan and cook for a further five minutes.

27. Garnish with coriander.

Pulled Pork

Pulled Pork is a versatile dish that can be used for just about anything such as added to salads, as a pizza topping (pizza base recipe in this chapter), or eating as is. There are no limits. Indulge in this delicious meal without feeling guilty. This recipe calls for a slow cooker. It could be made on the stovetop, but then you would have to keep an eye on it throughout the cooking period.

Time: 8 hours and 15 minutes

Serving Size: 6 servings

Prep Time: 15 minutes

Cook Time: 8 hours

Ingredients:
- 2.2 lb pork loin

- 4 large garlic cloves

- 1 apple

- 1 red onion

- 2 stems of rosemary

- 1½ tbsp sea salt

- 1 tsp onion powder

- 2 cups of bone broth or vegetable stock

- 1 tbsp molasses

- 1 tsp garlic powder

- 1 tsp dried thyme

Directions:
- Massage the molasses onto the pork loin.

- Remove the core from the apple and slice.

- Peel and halve the garlic.

- Peel and chop the onion into chunks.

- Add the bone broth or vegetable stock to the slow cooker.

- Add the onion, apple and garlic to the liquid.

- Add the dried thyme, onion powder, sea salt and garlic powder to a bowl and mix together.

- Rub the dry ingredients onto the molasses covered pork loin so that it is covered evenly.

- Carefully add the pork loin to the slow cooker.

- Add the rosemary to the pot.

- Cover and allow to cook for eight hours on low.

- After it is cooked, you can use a fork to pull the meat apart.

Seafood Chowder

There is no food that will bring you closer to a traditional fishing town like a hearty, wholesome Seafood Chowder. Normally cooked with fresh cream, vegetables from the nightshade family, and full of inflammatory agents which are sure to set your progress back. However, this recipe is full of flavor and has all the healthy benefits you need to keep your gut happy and healthy. The chowder can be cooked in bulk and portioned out to be frozen.

Time: 1 hour and 25 minutes

Serving Size: 8 servings

Prep Time: 25 minutes

Cook Time: 60 minutes

Ingredients:

- 2 large turnips
- 2 large sweet potatoes
- 1 large onion
- 2 celery stalks
- 2 large cloves of garlic
- 1 head of broccoli
- 8 oz of cod
- 28 oz muscles, cleaned and prepared
- 3 tbsp liquid coconut oil
- 1 tsp garlic powder
- 1 tsp onion powder
- 2 tbsp sea salt
- 1 tsp turmeric powder
- 1 tsp ground ginger
- 1 tsp ground cinnamon

- 1 can of coconut milk

- 2½ cups of bone broth, vegetable stock, or water

- Fresh dill.

Directions:

1. Turn the oven on to 350°F.

2. Wash, peel, and cube the sweet potatoes and turnips.

3. Wash and chop the broccoli.

4. Finely dice the celery.

5. Peel and finely chop the onion.

6. Peel and mince the garlic cloves.

7. Cut the cod into cubes.

8. Add the sweet potatoes and turnips to a large mixing bowl.

9. Add 1 tbsp coconut oil, sea salt, onion powder, garlic powder, turmeric powder, ground ginger, and ground cinnamon to the mixing bowl.

10. Stir to coat the sweet potatoes and turnips.

11. Place the sweet potatoes and turnips in a baking dish.

12. Cook for 25 minutes.

13. The sweet potatoes and turnips will not be cooked through at this point but will cook further when the seafood, vegetables, and liquid is added.

14. Add 1 tbsp coconut to a large saucepan and heat on medium.

15. Add onions and celery and cook for approximately five minutes until see-through.

16. Add garlic and mix around, careful not to burn.

17. Add the broccoli and the remaining salt.

18. Stir to combine.

19. Add bone broth, vegetable stock or water, and coconut milk to the saucepan.

20. Add the roasted sweet potatoes and turnips.

21. Bring the mixture to a boil.

22. Reduce the heat and allow it to simmer.

23. Cover the saucepan and cook on low for 10 minutes.

24. Add the mussels and codfish to the saucepan.

25. Cover and cook for five minutes.

26. Add the dill and stir.

AIP Spin on Takeout Favorites

Cauliflower Pizza Base

Everyone has their own preferences when it comes to pizza. For this recipe, you will have a pizza base that you can assemble with whatever you prefer without the guilt.

Time: 45 minutes

Serving Size: 1 serving

Prep Time: 20 minutes

Cook Time: 25 minutes

Ingredients:

- ½ a head of cauliflower
- ½ tsp garlic powder
- ½ tsp onion powder
- ½ tsp dried oregano
- 3 tbsp arrowroot flour
- 1 tbsp olive oil
- Sea salt to taste

Directions:

1. Wash and roughly chop the cauliflower.

2. Add to the food processor and blend until fine.

3. Put the cauliflower into a microwave-safe dish and partially cover.

4. Cook on high for approximately five to six minutes.

5. Remove from the microwave and turn the cauliflower onto a clean kitchen towel or muslin cloth.

6. Leave to cool.

7. When cool, squeeze out as much liquid as possible.

8. Return the cauliflower to a clean bowl.

9. Add arrowroot flour, garlic powder, onion powder, sea salt, dried oregano, and olive oil.

10. Mix until your mixture resembles dough.

11. Line a baking tray with parchment paper.

12. Turn dough onto the tray and shape it into the shape of a pizza.

When you have decided on your toppings, place your pizza base in the oven that has been preheated at 350°F. Bake your pizza base for 20 minutes. When removed, dress your pizza.

Topping suggestions

- Hey Pesto
- Hamburger
- Pineapple
- Pulled Pork
- Turkey
- Mushrooms (cooked)

The options are endless. Do not be afraid to be creative.

Sticky Pork Ribs

Time to put on the bibs and get messy. Eat like nobody's watching you. Lick your fingers without being eye-balled. Block out your surroundings as you indulge in this roadhouse favorite. This guilt-free, nutritious meal will have you coming back for seconds and thirds. Pair it with the No-Fuss Mayo, Dairy-Free Tzatziki, Cauliflower Dip, or Dairy-Free Yogurt.

Time: 6 hours and 40 minutes

Serving Size: 6 servings

Prep Time: 10 minutes

Cook Time: 6 hours and 30 minutes

Ingredients:
- 3 lb pork back ribs

- ½ cup bone broth, vegetable stock, or water

- Sea salt to taste

Sticky Glaze
- 6 tbsp honey

- ½ cup plus 3 tbsp of coconut aminos

- 6 large cloves of garlic

- 1 tbsp ground ginger

- ¼ cup of freshly squeezed lime juice

Directions:

1. Turn the oven on to 400°F.

2. Place the rack ribs on a clean surface with the bone side up.

3. Inspect the rack of ribs to see if there is a silver membrane on the ribs.

4. If you do see a silver membrane, it will need to be removed. This will prevent the ribs from curling up when cooked or being tough.

5. With a sharp knife, aim the tip below the silver membrane by the bones and make an incision.

6. Feel for the membrane.

7. Pull the membrane away from the bone.

8. Discard the membrane.

9. Line a baking tray with aluminum foil or parchment paper.

10. Cut the ribs into single portions.

11. Season the ribs with salt and place them on the baking tray.

12. Place the baking tray in the preheated oven and cook for 15 minutes.

13. Turn them over and cook for a further 15 minutes.

14. Add the bone broth to the crockpot.

15. Stack the ribs in the crockpot and cook on low for six hours.

16. The Glaze

17. Preheat the oven to 400°F.

18. Add the honey to a saucepan.

19. Add the coconut aminos, lime juice, garlic, and ginger to the blender.

20. Blend until you have a marinade.

21. Add the marinade mixture to the saucepan and bring to a simmer on medium-high heat.

22. Stir frequently. The marinade will thicken and become darker in color.

23. When reduced, the mixture will coat the back of a spoon.

24. When ready, remove the saucepan from the heat.

25. Line the baking tray with clean aluminum foil.

26. Remove the ribs from the crockpot and place them in a large bowl.

27. Pour the glaze into the bowl and stir to coat the ribs.

28. Place on the baking tray and into the oven.

29. Cook until the glaze starts to bubble and caramelize.

30. Remove from the oven and serve immediately.

Chicken Wings

Another favorite that is guaranteed to hit the sweet spot. Chicken Wings can be enjoyed as an appetizer or a main meal. Your tastebuds will be eternally grateful. This is an ideal party snack or a dinner party meal. The choice is yours as to how you would like to introduce your friends to your version of chicken wings. They will not believe you when you tell them that this lip-smacking recipe is free of all the ingredients that will cause an uproar in your intestines. You could always keep this little revelation a secret and wait for the verdict.

Time: 30 minutes

Serving Size: 4 servings

Prep Time: 5 minutes

Cook Time: 25 minutes

Ingredients:

- 12 chicken wings

- 2 tbsp honey

- ¼ cup of coconut aminos

- 2 tsp olive oil

- 2 tsp ginger paste

- 2 tsp garlic paste

- Sea salt

- Fresh cilantro

Directions:

1. Turn the oven on to 355°F.

2. Rinse the chicken wings and pat dry.

3. Line a baking tray with aluminium foil.

4. Place wings on the baking tray.

5. Sprinkle with salt.

6. Place the baking tray in the preheated oven and bake for 15 minutes.

7. Add honey, olive oil, coconut aminos, ginger paste, and garlic paste to a bowl and whisk together.

8. Remove the chicken wings from the oven.

9. Using a basting brush, coat the wings with the marinade.

10. Return to the oven and bake for 5 minutes.

11. Remove the baking tray from the oven.

12. Increase the heat.

13. Coat the wings with the marinade.

14. Return the baking sheet to the oven and cook for another 5 minutes.

15. Remove from the oven, and transfer the chicken wings to a serving dish.

16. Garnish with cilantro.

Dinner Extras

No-Fuss Mayo

Everyone likes a sauce or something familiar that has been eliminated from their diets. Mayonnaise is no exception. This creamy condiment is an excellent accompaniment for salads or as a dipping sauce for vegetable fries. Guilt-free with the right amount of tang.

Time: 5 minutes

Serving Size: 1 serving

Prep Time: 5 minutes

Cook Time: No cooking time

Ingredients:

- ⅔ cup of coconut oil

- ⅔ cup of avocado oil

- ½ tsp pink Himalayan salt to taste

- 2 tsp freshly squeezed lemon juice

- Pinch of garlic powder

Directions:

1. Add olive oil and coconut oil to a 16 oz mason jar.

2. Add the lemon juice, pink Himalayan salt, and garlic powder.

3. Using a hand-held immersion blender, blend the ingredients ensuring that all the ingredients are incorporated.

4. Mix for approximately one minute or until it is a fluffy and creamy consistency.

Twisted Barbeque Sauce

Aptly named the Twisted Barbeque Sauce because it looks like the regular barbeque sauce but with none of the original ingredients that would not be beneficial to your body. This version is gut-friendly, with less sugar and more natural goodness. Ideal for those Chicken Wings or with your Homemade Sausage burgers.

Time: 40 minutes

Serving Size: 6 servings

Prep Time: 10 minutes

Cook Time: 30 minutes

Ingredients:

- 1 tbsp freshly squeezed lemon juice

- 1 tbsp apple cider or red wine vinegar

- 1 tsp ground ginger

- ¼ cup of maple syrup

- 1 tbsp of rendered bacon fat

- 2 large carrots

- 1 large onion

- 1½ cups of fresh strawberries

- ½ tsp sea salt

Directions:

1. Wash, peel, and dice the carrots.

2. Peel and dice the onion.

3. Wash and chop the strawberries.

4. Add maple syrup, apple cider or red wine vinegar, ground ginger, carrots, onions, strawberries, bacon fat, and lemon juice to a saucepan.

5. Bring the ingredients to a boil over medium high heat.

6. Stir and reduce temperature to allow it to simmer.

7. Add salt and stir to dissolve.

8. Taste test to determine if more salt is needed.

9. Simmer over a low heat for approximately 20 minutes or until the carrots are soft.

10. Pour the mixture into the blender, careful not to get hot liquid on you.

11. Blend until a smooth consistency, approximately two minutes.

12. Return the mixture to the saucepan and simmer for approximately 10 minutes.

13. Remove from the heat and allow to cool.

14. When the sauce has cooled down, transfer to a mason jar or an airtight container.

15. Store in the refrigerator for up to five days, or can be frozen.

Cauliflower Dip

This creamy dip is an ideal accompaniment to have as a side for any meal, or as a topping for your pizza. No excuses are needed to use this dip with any meals featured across the breakfast, lunch or dinner chapters.

Time: 40 minutes

Serving Size: 2 servings

Prep Time: 10 minutes

Cook Time: 30 minutes

Ingredients:

- ½ a head of cauliflower

- 3 garlic cloves

- 3 tbsp olive oil

- 2 tbsp freshly squeezed lemon juice

- Sea salt

Directions:

1. Turn the oven to 400°F.

2. Wash and break the cauliflower into florets.

3. Add the cauliflower florets to a large bowl and add 2 tbsp of olive oil.

4. Stir to coat the cauliflower.

5. Turn the oiled cauliflower onto a lined baking tray.

6. Using aluminium foil, make a little parcel and add the unpeel garlic cloves and secure to ensure air does not escape.

7. Place the aluminium parcel on the tray.

8. Place the baking tray in the preheated oven and roast for 30 minutes.

9. Stir the cauliflower around halfway through the roast.

10. Remove the baking tray from the oven, cauliflower should be caramelized and soft.

11. Transfer the roasted cauliflower to the food processor.

12. Open the aluminum parcel, careful not to burn, and gently squeeze the garlic from the peel.

13. Add the garlic to the food processor.

14. Add freshly squeezed lemon juice and remaining olive oil.

15. Blend until the consistency represents a smooth puree.

16. Salt to taste.

17. Store in an airtight container in the refrigerator.

Chapter 12:

AIP Diet: Snacks and

Desserts

The wait is over. The chapter you have been waiting for is here. Here you will find a collection of sweet and savory delights to satisfy most cravings. By now you have been introduced to a lot of ingredients you never knew existed. You have seen the impossible become possible. Use what you have learned over the previous three chapters and experiment. If your experiment flops, try again.

Most of the recipes I came across said they were AIP appropriate, but when scrutinizing the ingredients, they featured ingredients that are not elimination phase friendly. Normally substitutes would be used to adapt the recipes but they would not end up with the desired results. It is important to read the ingredients of all recipes and compare them to your AIP food guide lists. Your health is more important than trying to undo all you have done to get to the point where your disorder is under control.

Enough babbling, let us get to the good, better, and best part of this book!

Sweet Delights

Guilt-Free Chocolate Cake

It might not be possible to imagine anything related to chocolate being guilt-free. Looking at the name sends alarm bells to your intestines in preparation for what is to come. Do not fear, this recipe was designed to keep your intestines happy, and keep you on the road to healing.

Time: 2 hours

Serving Size: 9 slices

Prep Time: 30 minutes

Cook Time: 30 minutes

Cooling Time: 1 hour

Ingredients:

Cake Mixture

- 3 ripe bananas

- 1 cup of pumpkin puree or mashed avocado

- 1 cup of sugar-free applesauce

- ¼ cup of liquid coconut oil

- 1 cup of cassava flour

- ½ cup of carob powder

- 1 tsp baking soda

- ½ tsp salt

Chocolate Frosting

- ½ cup of softened palm oil shortening

- ½ cup of carob powder

- ¼ cup of arrowroot flour

- ½ cup of coconut cream

- ¼ cup of honey

- ½ tsp of vanilla powder

- ⅛ tsp of fine sea salt

Directions:

1. Turn on the oven to 350°F.

2. Add mashed bananas, pumpkin puree or mashed avocado, applesauce, and coconut oil to a large mixing bowl.

3. Whisk to combine.

4. Add carob powder, cassava flour, baking soda, and salt to a small bowl and mix to combine.

5. Add the dry ingredients to the wet ingredients and mix well to combine and ensure that there are no lumps.

6. Pour the batter into an 8-inch square casserole oven dish.

7. Put the dish into the preheated oven.

8. Bake for 30 minutes.

9. Use a skewer or knife to see if the cake has cooked through. If not ready, bake for an additional 5 minutes until the skewer or knife comes out clean.

10. Remove from the oven and let it cool for an hour.

Chocolate Frosting

1. Add all the chocolate frosting ingredients to a large mixing bowl.

2. Combine the ingredients by using an electric mixer until smooth.

Assembly

1. Once the cake has cooled down, spread the frosting evenly over the top using a spatula.

Strawberry Goodness

Strawberries are a summertime fruit that have endless possibilities. We have seen strawberries being used in the Twisted Barbecue Sauce, you can make smoothies, and you can make pies. Yes, this is a delicious strawberry pie that will entice you into finishing the whole dish, but everything in moderation.

This recipe calls for a pie crust. You can use the gluten-free pie crust recipe from the Juicy Gluten-Free Chicken Pie (Chapter 10). Line your round baking dish with the pie crust, prick the base with a fork, and bake at 400°F for 20 to 25 minutes.

Time: 4 hours and 40 minutes

Serving Size: 8 slices

Prep Time: 20 minutes

Cook Time: 20 minutes

Resting Time: 4 hours

Ingredients:

- 3 cups of fresh strawberries

- 3 tbsp gelatin granules

- ¾ cup of water

- 2 tbsp apple cider vinegar and 4 tbsp water

- 1 cup of honey

- 3 tbsp arrowroot powder

- Mint leaves

Directions:

1. Wash and cut the strawberries into halves or quarters.

2. Add 1 cup of strawberries to the blender and puree.

3. Arrange the remaining strawberries in your prepared pie crust.

4. Sprinkle the gelatin granules into the water and mix to combine.

5. Add the strawberry puree, apple cider vinegar and water, and honey to a saucepan.

6. Heat on medium until boiling, while stirring.

7. Reduce the heat to low and allow to simmer until thickened, approximately five minutes.

8. Remove from the heat.

9. Add gelatin mixture and arrowroot powder to the saucepan.

10. Whisk to combine.

11. Pour the mixture over the strawberries in the pie dish.

12. Place your pie dish in the refrigerator for approximately four hours, or until set.

13. Garnish with mint leaves.

Lemon Jello

Light and full of natural goodness. Jello is the perfect dessert after any meal, as it will slide in and around so as not to take up more space in your stomach than is necessary. No need to undo the buttons of your shirt or pants.

Time: 4 hours and 14 minutes

Serving Size: 12 to 15 squares depending on the size of you dish

Prep Time: 10 minutes

Cook Time: 7 minutes

Resting Time: 4 hours

Ingredients:

- 1½ cups of filtered water

- ½ cup of freshly squeezed lemon juice

- 2 tbsp gelatin granules

- 2 tbsp honey

Directions:

1. Add freshly squeezed lemon juice and water into a saucepan.

2. Spring the gelatin over the top of the lemon and water.

3. Whisk the liquid to combine the gelatine and allow to rest for three minutes.

4. Heat the mixture on medium-low until the gelatin has dissolved.

5. Remove from the heat and add the honey.

6. Stir continuously until the honey has dissolved.

Guilt-Free Chocolate Mousse

Light and refreshing without the guilt. Can be enjoyed after a meal, at dinner parties, or at Christmas lunch. Whoever said diets were dull and bland need to come and try these recipes! Before starting this recipe, put your can of coconut cream in the refrigerator to chill for at least eight hours, or longer.

Time: 2 hours and 13 minutes

Serving Size: 4 servings

Prep Time: 10 minutes

Cook Time: 3 minutes

Resting Time: 2 hours

Ingredients:

- 1 can of full-fat coconut cream

- 18 dates, pits removed

- 2 tbsp carob powder

- ½ tsp vanilla powder

- 3 tbsp coconut oil

- ⅛ tsp of sea salt

Directions:

1. Remove the solidified coconut cream and all but ⅓ of the remaining water.

2. Add the cream to a saucepan.

3. Heat over low heat until the cream has melted.

4. Remove from the heat.

5. Add the dates, carob powder, vanilla powder, coconut oil, and salt to the blender.

6. Mix until a smooth consistency.

7. Pour into your containers of choice.

8. Place in the refrigerator for up to two hours until firm.

9. Serve with fresh berries or a spoonful of Dairy-Free Yogurt.

Banana Ice Cream Surprise

What would a dessert section of a recipe compilation be without ice cream? Ice cream is, after all, a favorite treat. Rain, snow, sun, or wind, everyone needs some ice cream in their lives.

Time: 5 minutes

Serving Size: 2 servings

Prep Time: 5 minutes

Cook Time: No cooking time

Ingredients:

- 6 frozen bananas cut into pieces.

- ¼ tsp vanilla powder

- ½ cup of unsweetened shredded coconut

Directions:

1. Add the frozen banana pieces into a blender.

2. Blend until smooth.

3. Do not blend too long, you do not want to melt the bananas.

4. Add shredded coconut and vanilla powder to the bananas.

5. Blitz for 30 seconds until combined.

6. Serve immediately.

Savory Treats

Gluten-Free Crunch

If you really do not have a sweet tooth, and you prefer a crunchy snack before bed, or any time of the day, you have stumbled on the perfect recipe. This recipe has the right amount of crunch into making you believe you are eating a bag of processed crisps. Use any of our accompanying dips or sauces to enjoy this guilt-free snack.

Time: 30 minutes

Serving Size: 2 servings

Prep Time: 10 minutes

Cook Time: 20 minutes

Ingredients:

- ⅓ cup of arrowroot flour

- ⅓ cup of cassava flour

- 4 tbsp cold water

- 3 tbsp olive oil

Directions:

1. Turn the oven on to 400°F.

2. Add the arrowroot flour, cassava flour, olive oil and cold water in a mixing bowl.

3. Mix well to combine all the ingredients and form a dough.

4. Line a baking tray with parchment paper.

5. Turn the dough out onto the baking tray and spread evenly across the baking tray with a rolling pin or spatula, consistency dependent.

6. Place the baking tray in the preheated oven and bake for approximately 15 minutes.

7. Keep an eye on the oven to make sure your dough does not burn.

8. Remove from the oven.

9. Break into bite-size pieces.

10. Allow to cool before eating.

11. Can be stored in an airtight container.

Herb Plantain Crackers

These crackers are an excellent addition to the snack table at a party. No need to stand around and watch how your guests are enjoying snacks while you are trying desperately not to indulge in all the "forbidden fruit". Make a couple of batches at a time and take a container to your next party. Do not forget your dips. Be prepared to share your recipe.

Time: 1 hour and 15 minutes

Serving Size: 2 servings

Prep Time: 15 minutes

Cook Time: 1 hour

Ingredients:

- 2 large plantains

- 2 tbsp of freshly chopped rosemary

- 1 tsp garlic powder

- ½ tsp sea salt

- ½ cup of coconut oil

Directions:

1. Turn the oven on to 300°F.

2. Cut and peel the plantains.

3. Chop them up roughly and put in the blender.

4. Add rosemary, garlic powder, sea salt, coconut oil into the blender with the plantains.

5. Blend until a chunky mixture forms.

6. Line your baking tray with parchment paper.

7. Turn the mixture from the blender onto the baking tray.

8. Spread evenly over the baking tray with a spatula or rolling pin, approximately ¼-inch thickness.

9. Place in the preheated oven for 1o minutes.

10. Remove from the oven and cut into bite-size shapes.

11. Return to the oven and cook for approximately 50 minutes.

12. The end product will have a medium brown color and not soft to the touch.

13. Cook in increments of 10 minutes until you are satisfied with the crispness.

14. Remove from the oven when ready and allow to cool.

15. Break the crackers apart along the lines you created at the beginning of the cooking time.

16. Store in an airtight container.

Crispy Pork Rinds

If you have not tried pork rinds before, now is the time to tickle the taste buds and get acquainted with a delicious crunch. It is gluten- and carb-free, it has got the right amount of healthy fats you need, and when prepared, has the crunchiest crunch you have ever had. You might end up reaching for your partner's share.

Time: 2 hours and 35 minutes

Serving Size: 30 to 50 pieces

Prep Time: 20 minutes

Cook Time: 2 hours and 15 minutes

Ingredients:

- 1 large slab of pork skin

- Sea salt

Directions:

1. Turn your oven on to 250°F.

2. Lay the pork skin on a clean surface.

3. Remove the fat from the skin. Do not discard the fat, use it to make lard by adding it to a large saucepan and cooking over low heat.

4. When you have removed the fat, slice the skin into small pieces.

5. Sprinkle with salt, a generous helping.

6. Put the skin on a cooling rack, over a baking tray.

7. Put the baking tray in the preheated oven and bake for approximately two hours. It should be dried out at this point.

8. Remove from the oven.

9. Increase the heat to 400°F.

10. Move the skins to a clean cooling rack and baking tray.

11. Return to the oven and bake for approximately five to 10 minutes. The skin will begin to blister and crackle.

12. Remove from the oven and allow to cool completely before placing in an airtight container.

Optional

- You can season your pork rinds with any AIP-friendly herbs and spices.

Onion Ring Special

This recipe can be used as part of a meal or enjoyed as a standalone snack. Onion rings are a favourite, alongside fries, at all steakhouses. Eat it as is, or dunk it in your Twisted Barbeque Sauce. You better make a double batch because you will not want to stop once you start.

Time: 15 minutes

Serving Size: 2 servings

Prep Time: 5 minutes

Cook Time: 10 minutes

Ingredients:

- 1 medium-sized onion

- 2.8 oz of pork rinds

- 1 tbsp gelatin granules

- 3 tbsp boiling water

Directions:

- Turn the oven to 425°F.

- Peel the onion.

- Slice the onion into rings, not too thin.

- Add the pork rinds to the blender and blend to form crumbs.

- Transfer the pork crumbs to a bowl.

- Add the boiling water to a small bowl and add the gelatin granules.

- Whisk briskly to dissolve.

- Dip your onion rings into the hot gelatin, and shake off excess liquid.

- Place the onion rings into the crumbs and coat well.

- Place on a cooling tray over a baking tray.

- Repeat the process until your onions are finished, or if the gelatin mixture and pork rinds are finished.

- Transfer the baking tray to the preheated oven and bake for approximately 8 minutes, rotating the tray once during this time.

- Remove the baking tray from the oven and allow to cool slightly before serving.

- Add salt to taste.

Note

If you find the coating process too difficult, you can use a sandwich bag. Transfer the crumbs to the bag and add the onion rings in batches, after being dipped, and shake the bag around to ensure even coating. Remove from the bag and place on the cooling rack.

Conclusion

You have been on a crazy rollercoaster ride. A ride that took you to unknown places where you learned stuff you might have heard but dismissed as being hearsay. A ride that made you stand back and think about what you are doing. A ride that was filled with terminology you might never have heard of. A peek at some of the unseen issues people are faced with. A glimpse at what life could be like with the right self-care routine. A tour of a unique restaurant serving food that looks too good to be true. Yes, you definitely went on a rollercoaster ride.

The end is in sight, and you are either happy that it is coming to an end so that you can start reading from the start again, or trying to skip forward to see where the hidden chapters are. Whatever your reason is, I am happy that I got to ride alongside you on this adventure. I pride myself that I am in the position to share my knowledge with you. After years of research, and the world in the state it is today, it was the right time to reach out a hand to you.

Autoimmune disorders are real. We have learned that throughout this book. From the introduction to the conclusion, you have seen snippets referring to your health and well-being. While there are no cures for these disorders as yet, you, yes YOU, can make positive changes that can help stabilize your condition. While you make those positive changes and keep taking care of yourself, we will hope together that someday soon cures will be found.

Discovery

You got an up-close and personal view of what is going on inside your body. The things no one thought you needed to know. Thanks to this world in crisis, you heard words and you wanted to know what it all meant. You might have visited Dr. Google, and what you got in return was more questions than answers. You wanted clear and concise information that you would be able to understand.

The battle that is going on in our bodies on a daily basis is real. The battles happen in everyone who is alive and breathing. Some experience a little more negative love than others, and then a fight breaks out. We may even be so bold as to suggest that there are a lot of jealous antibodies that attack each other. That they want to be the only one protecting your body. Maybe the scientists should develop something to let the antibodies know that they should share. Jokes aside. The struggle is real. People suffer.

You were presented with a lot of different autoimmune disorders, and each came with symptoms. Some disorders presented the same symptoms, some of those symptoms are issues even healthy people are faced with. Do not ignore the symptoms. Every sniff, cough, sneeze, sore muscle, night sweats, or tingle in your fingers could be an early warning system. Visit your doctor if the symptoms are recurring. It might be nothing but it might also be something. You only have one life, so take care of it.

Food for Thought

You have been equipped with a toolbox to help you make the right choices. Use the Autoimmune Protocol to make positive changes. Changes that could help you or your loved ones. Being diagnosed with an autoimmune disorder is and should not be a death sentence. Allow yourself a day or two for a pity party, but pick yourself up and say that you are a good person, you have been a good person, and you will continue being a good person. You are your own worst enemy, and only you have the ability to change that around. Accept, adjust, and adapt to the new and improved you. Be the best that you can be.

The Time Has Come

It is now or never. Take the knowledge you have gained, take a giant leap of faith, and embrace the new you. Anything is possible when you believe in goodness. Look for the silver lining around every cloud, and keep on holding onto the belief that the doctors, researchers, and scientists are working hard on finding cures.

If you enjoyed this book, please leave a review on Amazon. Feel free to share your autoimmune disorder experience with your fellow readers, someone might be experiencing the same feelings you have. If you have any questions or suggestions, please leave a comment in the review section. The more you share about your experiences, the more it will help others understand what you are going through.

"I've seen better days, but I've also seen worse. I don't have everything that I want, but I do have all I need. I woke up with some aches and pains, but I woke up. My life may not be perfect, but I am blessed." — Unknown

References

AIDS.gov. (2015, August 11). *Organs of the immune system by AIDS.gov.jpg. Public domain.* Wikimedia Commons. https://commons.wikimedia.org/wiki/File:Org ans_of_the_Immune_System_by_AIDS.gov.jpg

5MinuteSchool. (2018). B Cells vs T Cells | B Lymphocytes vs T Lymphocytes - Adaptive Immunity - Mechanism [Video]. *YouTube.* https://www.youtube.com/watch?v=NMOH Wry8EDc

AIP lifestyle. (n.d.). *Autoimmune Paleo BBQ Sauce - Primal Palate | Paleo Recipes.* Primal Palate. Retrieved December 11, 2020, from https://www.primalpalate.com/paleo-recipe/autoimmune-paleo-bbq-sauce/

AIP Ramen Recipe from 30-Minute Meals for the Paleo AIP ebook. (2018, August 5). Comfort Bites. https://www.comfortbites.co.uk/2018/08/aip-ramen-recipe-from-30-minute-meals.html

Ashley, M. (2017, July 12). *Lemon Blueberry Muffins (AIP, Paleo).* Its All About AIP. https://www.itsallaboutaip.com/lemon-blueberry-muffins-aip-paleo/

Autoantibodies | Lab Tests Online. (n.d.). Labtestsonline.org. https://labtestsonline.org/tests/autoantibodies

Ballantyne, Dr. S. (2012a, August 23). *Beef Breakfast Sausage (AIP-friendly).* The Paleo Mom. https://www.thepaleomom.com/recipe-beef-breakfast-sausage-aip/

Ballantyne, Dr. S. (2012b, September 13). *Reintroducing Foods after Following the Autoimmune Protocol.* The Paleo Mom. https://www.thepaleomom.com/reintroducing-foods-after-following-the-autoimmune-protocol/

Ballantyne, Dr. S. (2016, September 3). *Shaved Brussels Salad.* The Paleo Mom. https://www.thepaleomom.com/shaved-brussels-salad/

Ballantyne, Dr. S. (2019, October 29). *The 3 Phases of the Autoimmune Protocol.* The Paleo Mom. https://www.thepaleomom.com/the-3-phases-of-the-autoimmune-protocol/

Ballantyne, Dr. S. (n.d.). *What is The Autoimmune Protocol—The Paleo Mom.* The Paleo Mom; The Paleo Mom. https://www.thepaleomom.com/start-here/the-autoimmune-protocol/

Bell, B. (2017, February 2). *Is Leaky Gut Syndrome a Real Condition? An Unbiased Look.* Healthline; Healthline Media. https://www.healthline.com/nutrition/is-leaky-gut-real

Beth. (2019, December 28). *What is the AIP lifestyle?* Bon Aippetit. https://bonaippetit.com/what-is-the-aip-lifestyle/

Bryant, R. (2017, June 14). *Classic Dairy Free Tzatziki.* Meatified. https://meatified.com/classic-dairy-free-tzatziki/

Bryant, R. (n.d.). *Sweet & Salted AIP Granola.* Meatified. Retrieved December 5, 2020, from https://meatified.com/sweet-salted-aip-granola/

Carteron, N. (2019, December 6). *Lupus: Causes, Types, and Symptoms.* Healthline. https://www.healthline.com/health/lupus

Chandrasekaran, A., Groven, S., Lewis, J. D., Levy, S. S., Diamant, C., Singh, E., & Konijeti, G. G. (2019). An Autoimmune Protocol Diet improves patient-reported quality of life in inflammatory bowel disease. *Crohn's & Colitis 360, 1*(3). https://doi.org/10.1093/crocol/otz019

Chen, B. (2019a, June 10). *Strawberry Pie.* Bon Aippetit. https://bonaippetit.com/strawberry-pie/

Chen, B. (2019b, October 9). *AIP Chocolate Cake*. Bon Aippetit. https://bonaippetit.com/aip-chocolate-cake/

Daniel, A. (2018, February 7). *40 Health Myths You Hear Every Day*. Best Life; Best Life. https://bestlifeonline.com/health-myths/

Definition of Autoimmunity & Autoimmune Disease — *Autoimmune Disease | Johns Hopkins Pathology*. (n.d.). Pathology.Jhu.Edu. https://pathology.jhu.edu/autoimmune/definiti ons

Definition: Autoimmunity (for Parents) - Nemours KidsHealth. (n.d.). Kidshealth.org. https://kidshealth.org/en/parents/autoimmuni ty.html

Dinse, G. E., Parks, C. G., Weinberg, C. R., Co, C. A., Wilkerson, J., Zeldin, D. C., Chan, E. K. L., & Miller, F. W. (2020). Increasing prevalence of antinuclear antibodies in the United States. *Arthritis & Rheumatology*, *72*(6), 1026–1035. https://doi.org/10.1002/art.41214

Dock, E. (2018, August 22). *Graves' Disease*. Healthline; Healthline Media. https://www.healthline.com/health/graves-disease

Erin. (2017, January 30). *Paleo Vegan Chocolate Mousse (GAPS, AIP-friendly)*. Texanerin Baking.

https://www.texanerin.com/paleo-vegan-chocolate-mousse/

Frankham, J. (2014, April 28). *The Galloping Gourmet's Trans-Tasman Root Vegetable Soup Competition...* Joannafrankham.com. https://joannafrankham.com/best-root-vegetable-soup/

gohealthywithbea. (2020a, August 23). *Beetroot carpaccio (AIP, paleo, vegan).* Go Healthy With Bea. https://gohealthywithbea.com/beetroot-carpaccio/

Graves' disease - Symptoms and causes. (n.d.). Mayo Clinic. https://www.mayoclinic.org/diseases-conditions/graves-disease/symptoms-causes/syc-20356240

Gunnars, K. (2019, May 28). *Omega-3 Fatty Acids- The Ultimate Beginner's Guide.* Healthline. https://www.healthline.com/nutrition/omega-3-guide

Haber, A. (2015, March 2). *Silky Sweet Potato Puree [AIP/Whole30].* Grazed & Enthused. https://grazedandenthused.com/silky-sweet-potato-puree-aipwhole30/

Hashimoto's disease - Symptoms and causes. (n.d.). Mayo Clinic. https://www.mayoclinic.org/diseases-conditions/hashimotos-disease/symptoms-causes/syc-20351855

Healing Family Eats. (2020, July 5). *Lamb and Dill Meatballs with Creamy Mushroom Sauce, Cauli Mash {AIP, GAPS, SCD, Paleo, Whole30}*. Healing Family Eats. https://healingfamilyeats.com/lamb-dill-meatballs-creamy-mushroom-sauce-aip/

Healthline Editorial Team. (2020a, May 8). *Inflammatory Bowel Disease: Types, Causes, and Risk Factors*. Healthline. https://www.healthline.com/health/inflammatory-bowel-disease

Healthline Editorial Team. (2020b, August 6). *Rheumatoid Arthritis: Symptoms, Causes, Treatment, and More*. Healthline. https://www.healthline.com/health/rheumatoid-arthritis

Healy, H. (2018, June 28). *Healthy Chicken Finger Recipe (Paleo, AIP & Keto)*. Healy Eats Real. https://healyeatsreal.com/chicken-finger-recipe/

Hendon, L. (2014, July 19). *Super Fast Paleo Smoked Salmon Salad Recipe*. Paleo Flourish. https://paleoflourish.com/super-fast-paleo-smoked-salmon-salad-recipe

Hendon, L. (2015, December 4). *The Ultimate AIP (Autoimmune Protocol) Food List*. Healing Autoimmune. https://healingautoimmune.com/aip-food-list

Hendon, L. (2016, August 18). *AIP Apple Cauliflower Porridge - Guest Post by Louise Hendon*. The Paleo Mom. https://www.thepaleomom.com/aip-cauliflower-porridge-louise-hendon/

Hendon, L. (2017a, February 1). *Asian Garlic Beef Noodles Recipe [Paleo, Keto, AIP]*. Paleo Flourish. https://paleoflourish.com/asian-garlic-beef-noodles-recipe

Hendon, L. (2017b, October 5). *AIP Loco Moco Burger*. Healing Autoimmune. https://healingautoimmune.com/aip-loco-moco-burger-recipe

Hendon, L. (2017c, October 17). *AIP Cauliflower Dip*. Healing Autoimmune. https://healingautoimmune.com/aip-cauliflower-dip-recipe

Hendon, L. (2017d, October 24). *AIP Cauliflower Pizza Recipe with Pesto*. Healing Autoimmune. https://healingautoimmune.com/aip-cauliflower-pizza-with-pesto-recipe

Hendon, L. (2017e, November 1). *AIP Waldorf Salad*. Healing Autoimmune. https://healingautoimmune.com/aip-waldorf-salad-recipe

Hendon, L. (2018a, February 26). *AIP Chili Con Carne*. Healing Autoimmune.

https://healingautoimmune.com/aip-chili-con-carne-recipe

Hendon, L. (2018b, May 14). *AIP Zucchini "Lasagna" Recipe*. Healing Autoimmune. https://healingautoimmune.com/aip-zucchini-lasagna-recipe

Hendon, L. (2018c, May 28). *AIP Waffles Recipe*. Healing Autoimmune. https://healingautoimmune.com/aip-waffles-recipe

Hendon, L. (2018d, June 3). *AIP Flatbread Recipe*. Healing Autoimmune. https://healingautoimmune.com/aip-flatbread-recipe

Hendon, L. (2018e, June 3). *AIP Tomato-Less Ketchup Recipe*. Healing Autoimmune. https://healingautoimmune.com/aip-tomato-less-ketchup-recipe

Hendon, L. (2018f, June 8). *AIP Coconut Lime Shrimp Recipe*. Healing Autoimmune. https://healingautoimmune.com/aip-coconut-lime-shrimp-recipe

Hendon, L. (2018g, June 11). *AIP Pork Rinds Recipe*. Healing Autoimmune. https://healingautoimmune.com/aip-pork-rinds-recipe

Hendon, L. (2018h, June 20). *Simple AIP Basil Pesto Recipe*. Healing Autoimmune. https://healingautoimmune.com/simple-aip-basil-pesto-recipe

Hendon, L. (2018i, September 9). *AIP Chicken Breakfast Casserole Recipe*. Healing Autoimmune. https://healingautoimmune.com/aip-chicken-breakfast-casserole-recipe

Hendon, L. (2018j, October 14). *Crunchy Paleo Crackers Recipe*. Paleo Flourish. https://paleoflourish.com/crunchy-paleo-crackers-recipe

Hendon, L. (2018k, November 18). *AIP Sweet Potato Hash Browns*. Healing Autoimmune. https://healingautoimmune.com/aip-sweet-potato-hash-browns

Hendon, L. (2019a, February 5). *AIP Chicken Wings Recipe*. Healing Autoimmune. https://healingautoimmune.com/aip-chicken-wings-recipe

Hendon, L. (2019b, February 20). *AIP Red Velvet Smoothie Recipe*. Healing Autoimmune. https://healingautoimmune.com/aip-red-velvet-smoothie-recipe

Hendon, L. (2019c, April 24). *AIP Baked Onion Rings Recipe*. Healing Autoimmune.

https://healingautoimmune.com/aip-baked-onion-rings-recipe

Hermes LDG. (2015, September 10). *Chicken roasting food – Free photo on Pixabay.* Pixabay. https://pixabay.com/photos/chicken-roasting-food-salad-dish-1618459/

Higuera, V. (2020, October 30). *What is Ulcerative Colitis?* Healthline; Healthline Media. https://www.healthline.com/health/ulcerative-colitis

Holland, K. (2020a, June 30). *Crohn's Disease: Causes, Symptoms, Diagnosis, and More.* Healthline. https://www.healthline.com/health/crohns-disease

Holland, K. (2020b, June 30). *Everything You Need to Know About Psoriasis.* Healthline; Healthline Media. https://www.healthline.com/health/psoriasis

Hoover, M. (2019, December 16). *Paleo Chicken Pot Pie (AIP).* Unbound Wellness. https://unboundwellness.com/paleo-chicken-pot-pie/

How your baby's immune system develops. (2019, June). Pregnancybirthbaby.org.Au; {{meta.dc.publisher}}. https://www.pregnancybirthbaby.org.au/how-your-babys-immune-system-develops

Immune system. (2019, May). Healthdirect.Gov.Au; Healthdirect Australia. https://www.healthdirect.gov.au/immune-system

Jay, K. (2016, April 20). *Baked Sweet Potatoes, with Sardines, Green Olives and Kale.* Autoimmune Wellness. https://autoimmunewellness.com/baked-sweet-potatoes-sardines-green-olives-kale/

Kivi, R. (2020, June 17). *Type 1 Diabetes: Symptoms, Treatment, Causes, and Vs. Type 2.* Healthline. https://www.healthline.com/health/type-1-diabetes-causes-symtoms-treatments

Kristina. (2018, March 14). *Homemade Coconut Yogurt {Vegan, Dairy-Free}.* Vibrant Plate. https://www.vibrantplate.com/homemade-coconut-yogurt-dairy-free/

Kubala, J. (2018, June 12). *Essential Amino Acids: Definition, Benefits and Food Sources.* Healthline. https://www.healthline.com/nutrition/essential-amino-acids

Kubala, J. (2019, August 8). *Food as Medicine: Does What You Eat Influence Your Health?* Healthline. https://www.healthline.com/nutrition/food-as-medicine

Kyle, E. (2019, November 5). *Bacon & "Eggs" + 20 AIP Breakfast Recipes.* Emily Kyle Nutrition.

https://emilykylenutrition.com/aip-breakfast-recipes/

Levey, D. K. (2018, January 22). *A Detailed Paleo Diet Food List of What to Eat and Avoid | Everyday Health.* EverydayHealth.com. https://www.everydayhealth.com/diet-nutrition/paleo-diet/detailed-paleo-diet-food-list-what-eat-avoid/

Lights, V. (2018, September 17). *Celiac Disease: More Than Gluten Intolerance.* Healthline; Healthline Media. https://www.healthline.com/health/celiac-disease-sprue

Lucia. (n.d.-a). *AIP Coconut Chicken Curry Recipe.* Alight with Healing. Retrieved December 6, 2020, from https://alightwithhealing.com/recipes/aip-coconut-chicken-curry

Lucia. (n.d.-b). *AIP Paleo Slow Cooker Pulled Pork Recipe.* Alight with Healing. Retrieved December 6, 2020, from https://alightwithhealing.com/recipes/aip-slow-cooker-pulled-pork-recipe

Lucia. (n.d.-c). *Seafood Chowder with Cod & Mussels Recipe.* Alight with Healing. Retrieved December 6, 2020, from https://alightwithhealing.com/recipes/aip-paleo-seafood-chowder-recipe

Manzel, A., Muller, D. N., Hafler, D. A., Erdman, S. E., Linker, R. A., & Kleinewietfeld, M. (2013). Role of "Western Diet" in Inflammatory Autoimmune Diseases. *Current Allergy and Asthma Reports*, *14*(1). https://doi.org/10.1007/s11882-013-0404-6

Mayo Clinic. (2018). *Crohn's disease - Symptoms and causes*. Mayo Clinic. https://www.mayoclinic.org/diseases-conditions/crohns-disease/symptoms-causes/syc-20353304

Mayo Clinic. (2019, March 1). *Rheumatoid arthritis- Symptoms and causes*. Mayo Clinic. https://www.mayoclinic.org/diseases-conditions/rheumatoid-arthritis/symptoms-causes/syc-20353648

Mayo Clinic. (n.d.). *Multiple sclerosis - Symptoms and causes*. Mayo Clinic. https://www.mayoclinic.org/diseases-conditions/multiple-sclerosis/symptoms-causes/syc-20350269

McCully, M. (2020, July 31). *Boosting immunity is a dangerous myth*. ELLE. https://www.elle.com/beauty/health-fitness/a33299126/boosting-immunity-is-a-dangerous-myth/

MD, A. M. (2016, July 29). *8 Autoimmune Disease Myths & Facts*. Amy Myers MD.

https://www.amymyersmd.com/article/autoim
mune-disease-myths-facts/

Medical Definition of SELF-ANTIGEN. (n.d.).
Www.Merriam-Webster.com. Retrieved
November 28, 2020, from
https://www.merriam-
webster.com/medical/self-antigen

MEDSimplified. (2020). Immune system made easy—
immunology innate and adaptive immunity
simple animation [Video]. *Youtube.*
https://www.youtube.com/watch?v=k9QAyP3
bYmc&t=245s

Nall, R. (2020, August 26). *Causes of Rheumatoid Arthritis.*
Healthline.
https://www.healthline.com/health/rheumatoi
d-arthritis-causes

Nemrow, S. (2020, August 20). *Autoimmune Protocol AIP
Maintenance Phase.* Shanna Nemrow.
https://shannanemrow.com/2020/08/autoim
mune-protocol-aip-maintenance-phase/

Nicole. (2020b, October 15). *Sweet Potato, Bacon and
Chive Muffins(AIP, paleo) • Heal Me Delicious.* Heal
Me Delicious.
https://healmedelicious.com/sweet-potato-
bacon-and-chive-muffins/

Petre, A. (2020, August 25). *AIP (Autoimmune Protocol)
Diet: Overview, Food List, and Guide.* Healthline.

https://www.healthline.com/nutrition/aip-diet-autoimmune-protocol-diet

Pfeffer, J. (2012, July 19). *21 Healthy Lifestyle Quotes to Inspire You | Rasmussen College.* Rasmussen.Edu. https://www.rasmussen.edu/degrees/health-sciences/blog/healthy-lifestyle-quotes-to-inspire-you/

Phillips, S. (2019, August 5). *Debunking 5 Autoimmune Disease Myths – Willow Integrative Wellness.* Willow Integrative Wellness. https://willowforlife.com/debunking-5-about-autoimmune-disease-myths/

Pietrangelo, A. (2017, January 24). *Guide to Lupus Symptoms.* Healthline. https://www.healthline.com/health/lupus/symptom-guide

Pietrangelo, A. (2020a, May 5). *Drinking Bleach Is No Cure for Coronavirus and Poses Serious Risks.* Healthline. https://www.healthline.com/health/drinking-bleach#will-drinking-bleach-kill-you

Pietrangelo, A. (2020b, May 15). *Everything You Need to Know About Multiple Sclerosis (MS).* Healthline. https://www.healthline.com/health/multiple-sclerosis

Pietrangelo, A. (2020c, August 6). *Early Signs of Rheumatoid Arthritis.* Healthline; Healthline

Media.
https://www.healthline.com/health/early-signs-rheumatoid-arthritis

Psoriasis - Symptoms and causes. (n.d.). Mayo Clinic. https://www.mayoclinic.org/diseases-conditions/psoriasis/symptoms-causes/syc-20355840

Rachael. (n.d.-d). *Sticky Honey Garlic Instant Pot Ribs.* Meatified. Retrieved December 11, 2020, from https://meatified.com/sticky-honey-garlic-instant-pot-ribs/

Resler, H. (2020). Createdelicious.com. https://createdelicious.com/paleo-cold-cereal-aip/

Robertson, R. (2017, June 26). *Why the Gut Microbiome Is Crucial for Your Health.* Healthline. https://www.healthline.com/nutrition/gut-microbiome-and-health

Samantha. (2016, March 17). *No-Mess No-Egg Mayo - AIP, Paleo, Whole 30.* The Unskilled Cavewoman. https://www.theunskilledcavewoman.com/no-mess-no-egg-mayo-aip-paleo-whole-30/

Spring, M. (2019, September 24). *Spiced Carrot AIP Breakfast Porridge.* Thriving On Paleo | AIP & Paleo Recipes for Autoimmune Disease Relief.

https://thrivingonpaleo.com/aip-breakfast-porridge-spiced-carrot-paleo-egg-free/

Spring, M. (2020, Summer 2). *AIP Cassava Flour Pancakes - Thriving On Paleo | Paleo & AIP Recipes*. Thriving On Paleo | AIP & Paleo Recipes for Autoimmune Disease Relief. https://thrivingonpaleo.com/aip-cassava-flour-pancakes/

Sunwell-Vidaurri, E. (2018, August 26). *Naturally Sweetened Homemade Lemon Jello*. Recipes to Nourish. https://www.recipestonourish.com/naturally-sweetened-homemade-lemon-jello/

Susan York Morris. (2018, September 28). *Everything You Should Know About Lymphocytes*. Healthline; Healthline Media. https://www.healthline.com/health/lymphocytes

The Immune System. (2019). Johns Hopkins Medicine. https://www.hopkinsmedicine.org/health/conditions-and-diseases/the-immune-system

Three Myths on Autoimmune Disease - Healthy options, Philippines : News Digest. (n.d.). Healthy Options. Retrieved November 30, 2020, from https://www.healthyoptions.com.ph/newsdigest/supercharge-yourself/three-myths-on-autoimmune-disease

Tiffany. (2015, June 18). *Banana-Coconut Raw Vegan Ice Cream*. The Coconut Mama. https://thecoconutmama.com/banana-coconut-raw-vegan-ice-cream/

Ulcerative colitis - Symptoms and causes. (2018). Mayo Clinic. https://www.mayoclinic.org/diseases-conditions/ulcerative-colitis/symptoms-causes/syc-20353326

Van Tiggelen, S. (n.d.-a). *AIP / Paleo Bacon-Wrapped Pears - Easy Appetizer Recipe*. A Squirrel in the Kitchen. Retrieved December 11, 2020, from https://asquirrelinthekitchen.com/aip-paleo-bacon-wrapped-pears-easy-appetizer-recipe/

Van Tiggelen, S. (n.d.-b). *What is the Paleo Autoimmune Protocol (or AIP)?* A Squirrel in the Kitchen. https://asquirrelinthekitchen.com/what-is-the-paleo-autoimmune-protocol-or-aip/

Watson, S., Lights, V., & Boskey, E. (2019, March 8). *Psoriatic Arthritis: Types, Symptoms, Diagnosis, and More*. Healthline. https://www.healthline.com/health/psoriatic-arthritis

Wellness, A. (2014, February 18). *Garlic Rosemary Plantain Crackers*. Autoimmune Wellness. https://autoimmunewellness.com/garlic-rosemary-plantain-crackers/

Wendi's AIP Kitchen. (2017a, September 30). *Butternut Squash Soup w/Lemon & Tarragon*. Wendi's AIP Kitchen. https://wendisaipkitchen.com/2017/09/30/butternut-squash-soup-wlemon-tarragon/#wpzoom-premium-recipe-card

Wendi's AIP Kitchen. (2017b, October 1). *The Richest Bone Broth (AIP/Paleo)*. Wendi's AIP Kitchen. https://wendisaipkitchen.com/2017/10/01/the-richest-bone-broth-aip/

What Causes Lupus? | Lupus Foundation of America. (n.d.). Www.Lupus.org. Retrieved December 2, 2020, from https://www.lupus.org/resources/what-causes-lupus#

Wint, C. (2019, August 15). *Hashimoto's Disease: Causes, Symptoms, and Treatment*. Healthline. https://www.healthline.com/health/chronic-thyroiditis-hashimotos-disease

Wyant, P. (2018, June 28). *12 Myths About Autoimmune Disease That Make It Even Harder to Live With*. The Mighty. https://themighty.com/2018/06/autoimmune-disease-myths-misconceptions/

CPSIA information can be obtained
at www.ICGtesting.com
Printed in the USA
BVHW041437200521
607797BV00001B/118